Lift

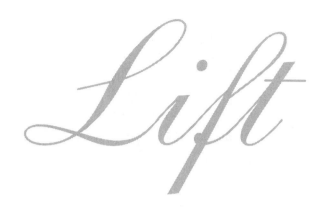

Lift

WANTING, FEARING, AND HAVING A FACE-LIFT

Joan Kron

Viking

guin Group
Hudson Street,
)014, U.S.A.
Vrights Lane,
London W8 5TZ, England
Penguin Books Australia Ltd, Ringwood,
Victoria, Australia
Penguin Books Canada Ltd, 10 Alcorn Avenue,
Toronto, Ontario, Canada M4V 3B2
Penguin Books (N.Z.) Ltd, 182–190 Wairau Road,
Auckland 10, New Zealand
Penguin India, 210 Chiranjiv Tower, 43 Nehru Place,
New Delhi 11009, India

Penguin Books Ltd, Registered Offices:
Harmondsworth, Middlesex, England

First published in 1998 by Viking Penguin,
a member of Penguin Putnam Inc.

3 5 7 9 10 8 6 4 2

Portions of this book appeared in different form in *Allure*.

Grateful acknowledgment is made for permission to reprint excerpts from *Full Gallop*
by Mark Hampton and Mary Louise Wilson, published by Dramatists Play Service.
By permission of the authors.

To protect identities, everyone quoted or described in this book by first name only (or by a letter of the
alphabet) has been assigned a fictitious name or letter. Those referred to by first *and* last names are either
public or historical figures, or people who have agreed to allow their real names to be used.

Visit Joan Kron's Web site at http://www.face-lift.com

LIBRARY OF CONGRESS CATALOGING IN PUBLICATION DATA
Kron, Joan.
Lift: wanting, fearing, and having a face-lift / Joan Kron.
p.   cm.
Includes index.
ISBN 0-670-87060-9
1. Face-lift—Popular works.   I. Title.
RD119.5.F33.K76   1998
617.5'20592—dc21   98–23436

This book is printed on acid-free paper.
⊗
Printed in the United States of America
Set in Deepdene
Designed by Jennifer Ann Daddio

For Linda Wells

CONTENTS

Before

1. HOW I GOT THIS FACE   1

2. IT'S NOT NICE TO FOOL MOTHER NATURE   9

3. LOSING FACE   23

4. FINDING DR. RIGHT   53

During

5. LIFE AND DEATH DETAILS   81

6. ANATOMY OF A FACE-LIFT   105

7. PRESSING OUT THE WRINKLES   139

After

8. PARDON MY APPEARANCE; I'VE JUST HAD A RUN-IN
   WITH A PLASTIC SURGEON   170

9. METAMORPHOSIS—THE BUTTERFLY EMERGES   205

10. IT'S YOUR DECISION   214

Check It Out   218

Acknowledgements   223

Notes   227

Index   257

One

HOW I GOT THIS FACE

"There are only two subjects worth talking about—menopause and face-lifts."
—A WASHINGTON NETWORK NEWSWOMAN, QUOTED BY GAIL SHEEHY,
IN *THE SILENT PASSAGE: MENOPAUSE*

I am older than Gloria Steinem and younger than Helen Gurley Brown. Until recently, when cameras became my enemy, I was certain I would never do it—have a face-lift, that is. In the 1960s, when I was in my thirties and married to a general surgeon, I went to a lecture on cosmetic surgery. "How horrible! I'll never have that," I exclaimed to the woman next to me, as graphic slides of a face-lift procedure flashed on the screen, taking me under the patient's lifted cheek flap and showing me all the tissue from her ear to her chin.

If those slides weren't a deterrent, my lumpy appendectomy scar was. "You can never have a face-lift," my mother warned. "You're like me, you're a keloid healer." She was operating under the common misconception that thick abdominal scars are keloids (they're not—keloids are cauliflowerlike tissue growths that spread beyond the bounds of the incision) and that a thick hypertrophic scar in one place on the body is predictive of how one will heal elsewhere on the body (wrong again—the face heals differently).

Like many women, I defused my feelings about aging by alternately joking about plastic surgery and condemning it. Deep down, though, everything about this rite of passage fascinated me—surgeon-shamans, secret-society membership, the scarification ceremony, cult of bravery, period of social withdrawal, and dramatic reentry with a younger visage.

Fast-forward to 1991. I am a journalist covering the psychology of appearance for *Allure* but I am still surprisingly clueless on the reality of lifts. I don't know the difference between a skin lift and a muscle lift, a phenol peel and a TCA peel. I can't tick off the names of the top plastic surgeons. All I know is that while I'm getting older-looking, many of my contemporaries are getting better-looking.

I finally had a reason to learn the ropes while on assignment in L.A., working on a piece about beauty rituals in the capital of self-invention. I scoped out the A-list of local surgeons and also discovered a uniquely Hollywood institution—the plastic surgery recovery house. On a tour of one of these pretty-in-pink establishments, I got my first look at women recuperating from face-lifts. Seeing one after another of these bruised, swollen-faced, tranquilized women was a sobering experience, especially when, in the middle of the house tour, a Beverly Hills Fire Department Emergency Unit arrived—siren wailing—in response to a 911 call about a postoperative patient who was hemorrhaging. I turned to the photographer working with me, rolled my eyes, and vowed, "Not me, ever."

So how was it that twenty-eight months later, I am in New York's premier plastic surgery facility—Manhattan Eye, Ear & Throat Hospital—as the bruised, swollen, tranquilized one in the helmet dressing, oozing bloody fluid through drains attached behind my ears. I have just undergone a two-and-a-quarter-hour face-lift (face, neck, eyes, and lip peel, to be precise) and my nonmedical second husband, a retired advertising executive, is standing at the foot of my bed, shaking his head and muttering helpfully, "You couldn't pay me to have this done."

When I assure him I'm feeling no pain and that considering the anticipated result, it's the most worthwhile discomfort I've ever endured, he thinks I'm delirious.

Within two weeks, his disbelief has turned to amazement. The swelling has subsided. I have graduated from Tylenol-and-codeine to plain Tylenol. The change in my appearance is remarkable. I am still myself, but a ten-years-younger-looking version of myself—the me I had lost. The result, I feel, is worth the temporary aches and annoyances— and, yes, even the money.

How do I explain this about-face?

Like many journalists, I have often used writing to work through my own personal issues. In fact, it was the death of my sixteen-year-old daughter in 1968 that propelled me into a writing career at the age of forty. I rescued myself from disabling sorrow by writing about grief therapy, and covering, for more than a decade, the emerging death and dying movement. When I divorced (as, I learned covering the field, many parents do after the loss of a child) and remarried, I had an identity crisis over what surname to use (second husband's name, first husband's name, maiden name?) and resolved it by writing about the legality of a married woman using a name other than her husband's. (I ended up keeping my first husband's name. I felt I owned it after using it for twenty years.)

And now I was ready to deal with another kind of loss: aging. It was through journalism that I started down the road to my first face-lift. *Allure's* editor, Linda Wells, expressed interest in having a first-person article on shopping for a face-lift. I volunteered, maintaining I was uniquely qualified. After all, I reasoned, I was one of the few writers in the room old enough to need one—not that I would ever want one.

The story required scheduling consultations with four leading plastic surgeons and *pretending* to want a face-lift. Undergoing one was *not* part of the assignment. The magazine would pay for the office visits, but not for surgery (and, of course, accepting any, gratis, in return for publicity was strictly forbidden).

Pretending turned out to be not that hard. I kept saying "it's just research," but with each visit, I became more open to the whole idea. I took to studying my face in the mirror and in old photos. Discussions with friends and acquaintances led to surprising confessions of trips to California for secret eye-jobs and face-lifts done literally under my nose. I was dumbfounded. If, as the handwringers say, a face-lift makes a person look like a test pilot in a wind tunnel, how come my friends had surgery without my realizing it? Obviously plastic surgery could be more subtle than I realized.

Sometime between the first phone call and the last office visit, I had crossed the line from stealth journalist to consumer. Impulsively I signed up for a $15,000 face- and eye-lift and lip peel—which is how I ended up in early 1992 in a bed in Manhattan Eye, Ear & Throat Hospital.

The magazine assignment that landed me in this hospital bed, "Shopping for a New Face," turned out to be more than a memoir of choosing a surgeon. It was also the story of my conversion. Afraid of jinxing myself, I had asked the magazine not to publish the article until after the surgery was successfully behind me. My literary agent, now deceased, advised me to have the lift and write about it if I wanted to, but not to use my own name. So, the piece ran a few months later under the byline "Anonymous."

To my surprise, the article struck a collective nerve. Letters and calls showed that, although I was older than the magazine's typical reader, the conflicting emotions I had experienced (grief for my lost youth, humiliation at the thought of possibly dying for vanity, sticker shock, confusion about the array of options, and my reluctance to grow old gracefully) were strikingly universal. Call it "growing old *dis*gracefully," but many people wanted to follow suit.

I'd given a lot of thought to choosing a doctor but little to the aftermath, specifically post-surgery protocol. It's customary after a face-lift, when people remark on your refreshed look, to credit your hairdresser or lie and deny—deceits that make me uncomfortable. Impulsively (again), I began telling the truth. If someone asked me why I looked younger, better, different, whatever, I usually said, matter-of-factly, "I had a face-lift." However, when a relative of my husband's ex-wife remarked bitchily, "I don't remember you being this pretty," I just smiled.

In return for my honesty, I was rewarded with an outpouring of confidences from women, and men, who were considering cosmetic changes and needed a sounding board. No matter how much you want it, the prospect of a face-lift evokes fear, shame, and embarrassment. Such superficiality calls into question your values about money, risk-taking, self-indulgence, and that most dreaded attribute—vanity. Perhaps the hardest thing about a cosmetic surgery purchase is admitting that you find something about yourself unacceptable, that you don't measure up, and worse, that you care. How uncool!

We want to believe it's what's inside that counts. But we know—from a lifetime of flattery, slights, deferential gestures, averted eyes, and other signs of approval and disapproval—that appearances count, too. We all have a back story. As a child, I was repeatedly told I looked like my father, not like my mother, who was often compared to the glamorous Sylvia Sidney. That hurt, but I got over it. Being talented was a compensation. I was never offered the ingenue role in the school play—and a good thing, because I suffered from terrible stage fright. I preferred to design the costumes. In college, studying theatrical design, I switched from Carnegie Mellon to the Yale Drama School because, at the time, Yale did not require designers to be in plays.

More recently, a friend told me that women like me (presumably, average women) cannot possibly understand how hard it is for women like her—very beautiful women—to lose their looks as they age. Gee, thanks. I have always had a sweet face. A little makeup, attitude, and a good haircut does wonders. I was much more concerned about my battle with weight than I was with my face. I never felt disadvantaged above the neck until I began to look in the mirror and see my grandmother.

I had hoped that a face-lift would make me recognizable to myself again and lift my spirits. And it did. It also gave me something I hadn't bargained for—a new career—or, more precisely, a new niche in my old career.

"Shopping for a New Face" launched me on the cosmetic surgery beat. I have traveled to Brazil to study the plastic-surgery star system; to Seattle to do a psychological autopsy on a dissatisfied patient who murdered her plastic surgeon and killed herself; to Hollywood to count the nose jobs of cosmetic surgery's most visible consumer, Michael Jackson; to Paris to visit the anatomy lab where important face-lift research was carried out in the 1970s; to Bologna to see where nose reconstruction surgery was perfected in the sixteenth century; and to a medical meeting in Orlando for the unveiling of the inconclusive first-year results of "the Twins Study": a shoot-out by four famous surgeons (sponsored by the University of California) to see which of four face-lift techniques yields the best results. Perhaps the most significant thing I've learned from all this is how far we will go in discomfort, expense, and risk for appearance. And how much justifying we do. Most people, I've found, believe *their* own face-work is absolutely necessary—and everyone else's isn't.

If you eventually have any, I warn you, once you've lost your innocence and had your first procedure—and it turns out well—you will very likely want more. Collagen and Botox injections often become a dress rehearsal for a face-lift. And one face-lift can occasionally lead to another, as I was to discover.

Nearly five years after my first lift, a recurring sinus condition required an operation. As long as I was having general anesthesia, I reasoned, why not have a few aesthetic adjustments on areas (brow and nose) I didn't deal with before. On the following pages, I'll be referring to my two trips to the "face factory" as my first lift and my second lift.

When I tell people I'm writing a book about the face-lift, they invariably ask me two questions. And as much as anything, this book is intended to answer them.

The first question: Are you "for" it or "against" it? Most people expect me to denounce it.

I stand, once again, somewhere between Gloria Steinem and Helen Gurley Brown, this time ideologically. (Steinem had an eye-lift, not to look younger, she has said, but in order to wear sleep-in contact lenses.) But she isn't opposed to cosmetic surgery for others if it is "life-enhancing." Brown, meanwhile, favors it wholeheartedly. (She has admitted having had a nose job when she was forty, a face-lift, and, more recently, an eye-lift and a mini face-lift.)

Obviously, I'm not against cosmetic surgery. What I am against is deciding to undergo it impulsively and signing up without being fully informed, or cutting corners on the doctor, the anesthesia, and the aftercare.

The second question, surprisingly: How old is the face-lift technique? There's a presumption that the operation is of recent origin, maybe thirty or forty years old, as if no one ever cared about their appearance or valued their youthful face before the self-involved "Me generation." Most people are surprised to learn that the first rhytidectomy, as it is called in medical parlance, was first attempted, timidly, in Germany almost a century ago, in 1901. But human beings have had relationships with their images ever since prehistoric people saw their reflections in bits of polished metal. Upper eye-lifts for, presumably, vision problems were performed in Imperial Rome in the first century and 1,000 years ago in the Arab world; and treatments to erase wrinkles and tighten sagging skin may date back at least 5,000 years and have been a constant since then, as has the debate about the virtue of beauty—having it, losing it, trying to get it back.

A recipe, written in hieroglyphs, for a rejuvenating acid face peel was found in the *Edwin Smith Surgical Papyrus*, circa 3000 B.C., the oldest existing surgical text. But, before you jump to conclusions about the time-lessness of female vanity, I should point out that the complicated instructions for preparing the paste and applying it are described under the headline: "For Transforming an *Old Man* into a Youth."

It's ironic. Here we are on the cusp of the twenty-first century. We have surgical remedies for the stigmata of aging that the Egyptians would have given all the gold in Tut's tomb for, and that Queen Elizabeth I, who, in her old age, outlawed looking glasses in her household, would have given the crown jewels for. Yet, we worry about the correctness of using the resources at our command. Having a face-lift isn't natural, critics carp.

But as *Times* health columnist Jane Brody pointed out recently in a column about another body practice that's considered "unnatural"—hormone replacement therapy: "A woman's current life expectancy, on average, of seventy-seven years is not natural either. Nature programmed us to live up to the age of menopause—long enough to bear children and raise them." What to do with our bodies and ourselves in these bonus years is the new dilemma.

In this book, I have tried to share some of what I have learned about the face-lift from history, from countless scientific presentations, and from talking to hundreds of individuals about their misgivings—and outcomes—and from my own surgeries. The most important lesson I can share may be that no two people have the same experience.

One woman is so ecstatic about her face work, she says, "I don't look at it as an expensive purchase. I consider it a new lease on life." At the other extreme is a self-described plastic surgery "victim," who went public on Sally Jesse Raphael's talk show. The disfigured patient is one of a small, but growing, number who fall into the hands of untrained and unethical practitioners. The woman's visage is every face-lift patient's worst nightmare. She has been advised she'll need six operations to correct her masklike appearance and over-operated-upon eyes.

But even when the quality of surgery is top-level, one patient can breeze through the recovery and her best friend can be miserable for weeks. Much like the experience of childbirth, there is no one standard kind of convalescence. The person who finds her first face-lift a breeze may find her second one a pain—and vice versa. The choice of doctor, your medical history, your attitude, your support system—all contribute to the outcome.

A face-lift is not for everyone. This book won't tell you whether or not you should have a lift, what doctor to go to, how much your surgery will cost, or what vitamins and herbal remedies to take beforehand. I'm always suspicious of writers who prescribe precise formulas. Each doctor has a preferred pre- and post-op regimen and there is no consensus except that aspirin before surgery causes bleeding and the so-called benefit of taking trendy Arnica is controversial. And, most of all, I can't promise a perfect outcome.

But, I hope, the book will help you clarify your attitude about the aging face and navigate between the mystery, the hype, and the old wives' tales surrounding restorative procedures. Friends can be a great support; however, as one surgeon warned, from his own experience, face-lift "patients receive notoriously inaccurate information from other patients who have undergone the procedure." Although several experts have reviewed the text for technical accuracy, this book isn't the last word on the subject. But I hope you'll find it to be a knowledgeable companion whether you're a serious candidate or just window-shopping.

Two

IT'S NOT NICE TO FOOL
MOTHER NATURE

[America] was founded on the revolutionary principle that [a person can not only]
make something of himself, he can make himself over.
—GILBERT SELDES, 1950

5:30 A.M. Tuesday. The Big Day. I'm due at the hospital in a half hour. After months of deliberation, consultation, justification, and preparation, I'm about to become one of the 90,000 (give or take) women to have a face-lift this year and one of a smaller number having a second one. I'm ready. I've cleared my calendar, paid my bills, stocked my refrigerator, made my excuses for my expected two-day absence, and taken two last snapshots—front and side view—to remember the way I am now. I've already filled my Vicodan prescription (a synthetic narcotic). There is, however, no prescription that can handle what I, having been through this once before, know is the most painful part of this experience: admitting to yourself and others that you want it and that you have voluntarily chosen it.

Actually, in my case, there are extenuating circumstances. No surprise there; there are always extenuating circumstances somewhere. My original reason for this trip to the hospital is that I can't breathe through my nose, so I'm having an operation to relieve a recurring sinus condition. This will be my third sinus repair in twelve years, and, according to several specialists, it may not be my last. Five surgeries in a lifetime is not unusual for this condition. I'm particularly apprehensive about my sinuses. My daughter died from a rare and virulent sinus infection contracted in Ceylon—now Sri Lanka—when my son, my daughter, and I accompanied my husband on a Project Hope teaching mission on the S. S. *Hope*, the hospital ship.

But I'm also pragmatic. Months ago, when a CAT scan confirmed the return of my sinus problem, I vowed not to undergo this surgery again without some *visible* improvement—and so arranged this doubleheader. After the otolaryngologist finishes with my nasal passages, a plastic surgeon (the same one who performed my first face-lift) will do a few "odds and ends," my euphemism for some not-minor facial procedures. Okay, I'm not the first cosmetic surgery patient to minimize the extensiveness of her surgery.

First comes an endoscopic brow-lift (a technique done through five tiny incisions in the scalp) to smooth out the scowl that's etched into my brow and makes me look angry when I'm not. There is a debate among doctors about whether the "endo brow" is superior to the traditional "coronal" browlift—but I'm willing to gamble to avoid the coronal's ear-to-ear scar across the top of the head and the hair loss and sensory disturbances it sometimes causes in the scalp. I have friends who have had successful coronal lifts. But I also understand that 35 percent of coronal brow-lift patients say they'd never have one again.

Next I'll have a tried-and-true TCA (tri-chloroacetic acid) peel on my upper lip to address those recurring lip pucker lines. For those of you who haven't mastered the vocabulary yet, I'll dissect the peel in chapter seven, "Pressing Out the Wrinkles." It may be trendier to have carbon-dioxide-laser skin resurfacing, and plenty of people find that method very effective, but I've heard too many reports of prolonged redness from that laser. I'm waiting for the new generation of gentler lasers. Until they're perfected, I'll stick with TCA. In fashion, it's fun to have the latest. In cosmetic surgery, I believe in waiting for the kinks to be ironed out of the technology and the practitioners to get further along on "the learning curve."

I'm also having a minor refinement of my nose. I saw a picture of myself in profile a year ago and was taken aback. My nose seemed to have grown longer and was tipping down like the Wicked Witch of the West. Doctors call it the aging-nose syndrome. Could this be addressed, I inquired of the plastic surgeon who did my original face-lift. Changing your nose, no matter how minimally, when you're an adult is risky business. The surgery is easy. But adjusting to even a slight change in a nose, no matter how much you desire the alteration, can be psychologically unsettling.

I suspect I was influenced by a doctor I interviewed once, who said, "If you change one feature, you get a small improvement, make two changes, you get a bigger one, change three things . . ." That remark stuck in my mind. I know it sounds irresponsible, perhaps even neurotic—could I be afflicted with body-dismorphic syndrome (the insatiable patient)? But I was curious about what a small change could make in my nose. One sign of post-modern society, says anthropologist Grant McCracken, "is our increasing curiosity about what the body could be and a willingness to tinker with it." I'm tinkering. And while we're at it, maybe we should revisit the face-lift.

There is no lifetime guarantee on face-lifts. One school of thought believes the longevity of a lift has to do with your age. The earlier you have it the longer it lasts—the later, the shorter. The other school says it has to do with your tissues. A recent study found that 5 percent of lifts relapse in one year. In any event, the best a lift can do is set back the clock several years, but it's going to start ticking again. If I weren't having the sinus surgery, I wouldn't be having a lift so soon after my first—but my doctor and I agreed the lift had begun to "relax" a bit, and he offered to give it a tug (or to "tweak" it, in the immortal words of Joan Rivers, who says she has something on her face "tweaked" every six or twelve months).

If I were seriously into recreating myself, I would have consulted a cranio-maxillo-facial surgeon (a specialist at reshaping the jaw and augmenting the skull). Changing the bone structure is really the only way to make significant physical alterations in a face. But that's not my goal or the goal of most women seeking rejuvenation. I don't want to change the topography, I just want to prune the trees—stop the skin, fat, and muscle from heading south.

My operative plan may sound extensive—but, after a certain age, there is a nagging fear that if you wait till next year or the year after, your internist will say, no surgery unless it's absolutely necessary. That's an interesting concept: necessary. A face-lift may not be a lifesaver in the traditional sense, but there's no question that, for many, it's a quality-of-life-saver, a lift in every sense of the word. Why else would so many accept the risks and the discomfort? Women today are having their first lift at ever younger ages, but for late adopters, like me, there's a now-or-never feeling. Longevity runs in my family and my nonagenarian mother has told me many times that she wished she had had surgery before she was too old to risk it.

I try to justify this venture as research, "participant observation" in ethnographic jargon—the same thing as Clinton Sanders, a University of Connecticut sociology professor, hanging out at tattoo parlors and having his arm covered with designs in order to study the cult of body alteration. Or Pat Moore, a young Columbia University student who disguised herself as "Old Pat," complete with gargle-induced raspy voice, and walked about in dozens of U.S. cities to observe the abuse and stigmatization of the elderly. Not incidentally, the few senior citizens Moore let in on the experiment confided they too felt like " 'young minds trapped behind old faces.' "

While beauty wasn't the goal, it occurred to me that looking a bit fresher wouldn't hurt on a book tour (even the *Times* made explicit, recently, what has been tacit for years: 'a beautiful visage often plays a role in how far an author gets'). Though there was always the chance I could look worse and be doomed by poetic justice to be a ghostwriter. But, like most patients, I felt the benefits outweighed the risks.

"Oh, face it," said a colleague, calling my bluff. "You want to have it."

Okay, I admit, I wanted it. The first lift was worth every penny. It was like having a makeover—only you didn't wash it off at the end of the day. My only regret after my first lift was not having done more. This trip, I'm taking care of the areas I neglected before. And though the surgery was used as research, my accountant told me, after it was over, "It is not tax-deductible. The IRS will say you had some personal benefit from it, and," he added, looking up from his calculator, "it's *obvious* you did."

Anyhow, back to my big day. I'm glad it's finally arrived. The anticipation is worse than the actual event. A friend told me that for weeks before her face-lift she had nightmares about emerging with a different face. During my countdown, I have woken up several mornings in a cold sweat with vague forebodings. Not being ill, I feel guilty for being melodramatic. A supportive call from my surgeon, acknowledging my apprehension, eased the tension on the last night. He assured me he was going to get a good night's sleep (or did I suggest it?). I always feel better after talking to him. Which, of course, is why I chose him in the first place.

Still, I didn't sleep well last night and worried I wouldn't hear my alarm. The hospital is conveniently around the corner from my apartment and I'm due there at 6 A.M. Having a face-lift in a hospital is no longer the norm, although I think it has benefits. Probably 70 percent of cosmetic surgery in the U.S. is performed in office surgicenters or in outpatient clinics run by doctors or hospitals. Proponents of outpatient surgery say that it's less costly and there's less chance of infection than in a general hospital. But because there may be no one looking over the doctor's shoulder, no committees, it's doubly important to check the credentials of the doctor and make sure the office is accredited—with all the necessary monitoring devices and emergency resuscitation equipment. (I'll talk more about this in chapter four, "Shopping for Dr. Right.")

My surgery is scheduled for 8 A.M. and I've had nothing by mouth since midnight. It's very important *not* to have food in your stomach when you're going to have anesthesia and lie flat on your back. Regurgitation of stomach contents can not only be unpleasant, but dangerous. But waiting around too long on an empty stomach can cause low blood sugar and make you light-headed. So, if you know your surgery won't start till later, you might try to negotiate a later deadline for halting food consumption. Whatever the time frame, don't overeat the day before in anticipation of a day without food. Since I've been doing hand-holding, I've noticed that many women get panicky at the thought of not eating for a day and try to compensate beforehand. Don't.

I've already bathed and washed my hair. I had my roots done two weeks ago, the last possible moment allowed by my surgeon (other doctors may be less strict). I was instructed to wear clothes that would be easy to get into for the return trip (nothing that goes over the head). And bring a big scarf and sunglasses to hide the bruising and the swelling.

Actually, this disguise won't fool anyone. It's like having a sign on your chest that says "I just had a face-lift," but trust me, you feel more comfortable in it.

I'm also bringing a robe for a stroll down the hospital hall the second evening. I'm staying two nights. The extra night adds another 300 dollars to my bill, but I think it's a worthwhile expense, since one complication, bleeding—though rare—tends to occur, if at all, in the first forty-eight hours. (Infection, a rare consequence, tends to strike a few days later.) I'm leaving my watch and wedding band at home. And I'm not wearing nail polish either, although bare nails are no longer a necessity for surgical patients. Before the introduction of the pulse oxymeter, which reads an anesthetized person's oxygen level, the anesthesiologist would watch the color of your nail bed to see if you were cyanotic—short of oxygen—a danger sign.

Which reminds me, I reviewed my will last night. It's fairly common to fear you'll be punished for your vanity. It's extremely rare to die from a face-lift, but having written about two women who did (one apparently didn't inform her surgeon or anesthesiologist that she had asthma, which may have contributed to her death; the other had a substance-abuse problem), I know I'm not just being melodramatic.

As one friend observed, "If you were rational you'd never put yourself under the knife." The idea of having one's facial skin peeled back, trimmed, tightened, and reattached sounds as barbaric as Chinese footbinding.

But social scientists know that large segments of society do not spend time and money and risk their lives on activities that do not serve meaningful goals. And that goal, contrary to what we've been told, is not vanity, says sociologist Kathy Davis, author of *Reshaping the Female Body.* Davis incurred the wrath of feminists when she took the position that cosmetic surgery "is not . . . imposed upon women." Many women see it, she says, as creating justice in a situation experienced as unjust—the unfair distribution of good looks and the unfair effects of aging. In view of the discomfort, expense and potential side effects, said Davis, women considering surgery spend a great deal of time deliberating and justifying, researching "the pros and cons, gathering information." The process helps them "put together their case" for surgery. They "may disapprove of it and at the same time desire it. . . . It's an ambivalent experience that needs to be explored."

Because of all the articles I've written on cosmetic surgery, I have become a magnet for plastic-surgery queries. Not only friends, but total strangers call me asking for advice, as if I know all the answers. I don't. I have learned to do more listening than advising—and this is what I hear. Curiosity. Desire. Apprehension. Ambivalence. These emotions are expressed to me every day by women—and men—who know that aesthetic surgery is my beat. "Cher was at the next table. She looks amazing. What did she have done and who did it?" . . . "What's the right age for the first lift? I hear you can't have it redone too many times or you start to looked pulled." . . . "How can I justify spending all that money on myself, when my kids could do so much with it?" . . . "A friend just had a face-lift. Her lip is drooping. Her doctor says it's temporary. I'd still consider having a lift, but I'd be so scared." . . . "Come on, tell me, who's the best?"

Wanting a face-lift is between you and your mirror. *Opting for one* is a political, moral, and social decision, often fraught with guilt, shame or, at the very least, embarrassment. Many women are as furtive about aesthetic procedures as they would be about abortion. I know young women who don't want their future husbands to know they've had their noses bobbed; women who deny their eye lifts to their best friends; and executives who won't tell their colleagues why they look so rested after vacations. Ten years ago it was estimated that 5 percent of the U.S. population has undergone cosmetic surgery to "erase signs of aging" or "move the recipient into the currently approved range of physical beauty."

That figure could be closer to 10 percent by now. There is no single source for cosmetic surgery procedural statistics. Several societies publish numbers based on polls of their own members. The figures used in this book, unless otherwise noted, are from the recent report published by the American Society for Aesthetic Plastic Surgery (an educational group representing 1,250 board-certified plastic surgeons): "ASAPS 1997 Statistics on Cosmetic Surgery." Not only ASAPS members were polled, but also those in other specialties (dermatology, otolaryngology, et cetera).

According to the survey, out of 2.1 million procedures performed in 1997, there were 99,196 face-lifts, 159,232 blepharoplasties (or eye-lifts), 55,000 brow-lifts, and 137,053 rhinoplasties. Skin treatments are going through the roof: chemical peels, 481,227; laser resurfacing, 154,153; dermabrasion, 40,214; collagen injection treatments, 347,168; Botox shots, 65,000.

Below the neck there were 176,863 liposuction cases; and—despite the negative publicity about implants—101,176 breast augmentations.

Women are still the biggest market (86.3 percent) for cosmetic work versus men (13.7 percent), except when it comes to surgical hair trans-plants (men have 50,566—five times more than women).

Women under thirty-five favor nose reshaping, liposuction, breast aug-mentation and reduction; women thirty-five to fifty increasingly attend to their faces, first resorting to eyelid surgery, chemical peels, and Botox and collagen injections before opting for the big-L, the lift. In the fifty-and-over group, face-lift numbers increase dramatically. With over 4 mil-lion baby boomers turning forty every year and marching reluctantly into middle age, and with 76 million baby boomers turning fifty—one every 7.5 seconds until the year 2014—and beginning, as The Wall Street Jour-nal predicted, "a very long old age," the cosmetic surgery ranks are bound to increase. That's a lot of secrets and lies.

Who can blame the secret keepers? Looking good is rewarded, but admitting you had help can carry a stigma. Hard-line feminists accuse cosmetic surgery patients of succumbing to male standards. Jurors in mal-practice cases, especially *female* jurors, are unsympathetic to patients who suffered injuries in the pursuit of beauty. It was only yesterday that physicians themselves thought of a patient seeking a face-lift as neurotic and in need of psychiatric evaluation. And at least one respected ethicist wonders if cosmetic surgery isn't a waste of social resources.

Class animosity lurks behind many of the digs at plastic surgery. When Gaspar W. Anastasi, a Boston plastic surgeon, was interviewed on a Toronto talk show, he recalls, "The first question was, 'How many Rolls-Royces are in your parking lot?' " The show's host assumed, mis-takenly, that all cosmetic surgery patients were wealthy. The same assumption was behind the Clinton administration's alleged consideration of a 100 percent luxury tax on aesthetic surgery, until one study reported that 65 percent of such patients had a household income of less than $50,000 a year. While Dolly Parton's surgery may get the headlines, Ms. America has become the real consumer.

The quest for physical perfection and an aversion to aging has been called "an American obsession." But sociologists believe it is a twentieth-century obsession that flourishes in capitalistic cultures where status is based on achievement rather than being ordained by birth. The French, once holdouts, are becoming rather knife-prone themselves, with more than 100,000 men and women out of a population of 58 million undergoing cosmetic surgery annually and having face work at a younger and younger age. Aesthetic surgery is sweeping the Middle East and Asia. Reuters reports that cosmetic surgery is a growth industry in post–civil war Beirut, where "nose jobs, cellulite reduction, breast implants, and face-lifts are fattening the bank accounts" of Lebanon's forty-some-odd registered plastic surgeons.

In India, thanks to the rising middle class, plastic surgeons can now earn as much as 7 million dollars annually. In South Korea, a recent study found, 35 percent of high-school and college students said they crave some kind of cosmetic surgery.

South American urbanites, of course, for decades have been way ahead of the U.S. in per capita consumption of cosmetic surgery. Nips and tucks are considered "permanent makeup" by Venezuela's beauty pageant participants. And in Rio, the typical Girl from Ipanema averages three beauty surgeries in her lifetime.

I'm not far behind.

5:50 A.M.

It's time to take a last look in the mirror. I notice that, without my eyeglasses, the lines and wrinkles are much less obvious to me. (Sitting in the dark was another of the aging Elizabeth I's solutions when she became "concerned with her vanishing looks.") The invention of spectacles is the perfect example of progress bringing unintended consequences. Sociologist Barry Glassner traces twentieth-century self-consciousness to the birth of the printing press. After its invention in 1451, wrote Glassner in *Bodies: Why We Look the Way We Do (and How We Feel About It)*, people began paying less attention to what they heard and more attention to what they saw, eventually becoming "more concerned about how they themselves looked." Nineteenth-century women believed the skin was the window of the soul. The development of photography heightened self-awareness. For Victorians, said Glassner, the rage for collecting photos of the rich and famous was the equivalent of our six-hour-a-day television habit. Those photos served as models for how to look and behave. With the advent of Thomas Edison's light bulb and better lenses, self-scrutiny soared.

By the end of World War I, wrote Ann Douglas in *Terrible Honesty: Mongrel Manhattan in the 1920s*, Americans dieted compulsively and weighed themselves obsessively on new Detecto bathroom scales. They measured everything from their IQs to their waists for the first-ever standardized clothing. Everything was seen with more clarity in their new eyeglasses. And not surprisingly, face-lifting took off in the 1920s.

World War I had a lot to do with it. The artillery caused wounds that had never been seen before and dentists and general surgeons devised techniques to fill gaping defects of the face and body. Bone grafting, cartilage transplants, artificial chins, progress in treating jaw fractures were just a few of the developments born of the Great War. Not to mention the speciality of plastic surgery itself. Before the war, there was only one general plastic surgeon in the U.S. and one in France.

There seemed nothing that imaginative surgeons couldn't do. A new genre of film plots about amazing transformations heightened that conviction. The subsequent development of safe anesthesia and antibiotics made it possible, at last, for individuals to alter their appearance with a minimum of pain and risk. And they wanted to more and more—and not just because of vanity.

The pressures of modern life—population mobility that made people from small towns strangers in big cities, social integration, women's liberation, the influence of mass media (especially film and later TV)—all contributed to the desire to look younger, more attractive, and less unusual. And new surgical techniques were the miracle stigma-removers.

It's possible that even the last disdainful holdouts will be driven to having surgery, defensively. According to *The Wall Street Journal*, the conversion in broadcasting in the next few years to High Definition Television (HDTV), a technology so unforgiving that every facial blemish looks like a moon crater, "will raise even higher the standards of pulchritude already prevailing in the industry," and "force broadcasters to hire even younger talent than they already do."

Not only the news anchors and talk-show hosts will be affected. A new self-consciousness will affect everyone from cooks promoting books to legal experts on Court TV, an outlet that is already said to have inspired more than one L.A. lawyer to have her face lifted before trying a high-profile case. With the advent of HDTV, one wonders whether the defendants will be having lifts too.

Today the public gets much of its plastic surgery information from television—the most influential medical journal in the world, if not the most accurate one. To keep queasy viewers from averting their eyes, or worse, switching channels, TV news-magazine producers build audiences with cosmetic surgery features, playing down the surgery and playing up the cosmetic results. Often procedures are made to seem as simple as a visit to the dentist for routine teeth cleaning. On *Donahue*, a doctor demonstrating a new wrinkle-erasing laser didn't wear a white coat and the patient didn't remove her earrings. On *20/20*, in a report dealing with a method of liposuction that can be performed using local anesthesia, a patient was shown talking nonchalantly on the phone while the doctor vacuumed fat from her hips. Little wonder that the day after these reports are aired, the featured doctors get an avalanche of calls.

The message is clear. Anatomy is no longer destiny. "People today view their bodies"—and other people's—"as increasingly malleable," observed sociologist Stuart Ewen in *All Consuming Images*. "The body is something that can be made and remade."

6 A.M.

Sleepy and a bit anxious, I wait with my husband to be formally admitted into the hospital. We are in an anteroom on the private floor where

I'll be recuperating. Another family group was here first—a woman who can't be more than forty and a couple I assume are her parents. Trying to be reassuring, the mother is gossiping about a friend who had a terrible face-lift. "It was done by some butcher in Florida," she says.

I imagine the daughter is recently divorced and getting a tune-up for reentry into the job market or the singles circuit. People often opt for cosmetic changes before or during "role transitions": new motherhood, divorce, remarriage, job promotion, a son or daughter's wedding, or a big birthday—especially ones ending in zero. "During such times of identity reconstruction," says marketing professor John W. Schouten, "people may be receptive to goods, services, or ideas that they formerly would have considered unnecessary or undesirable."

Come to think of it, my first lift coincided with the birth of my first grandchild. I joke that I'm not really a grandmother—just married to a grandfather, and there's a big-0 birthday in my future, too.

But inspiration can also come from the scary factoids on aging and demographics that are so frequently reiterated and replayed in the media. You've read them a hundred times. At the beginning of this century, life expectancy was 47.3 years. But in 1994, it was 75.7 years. The women will outlive the men but more women will live alone because widowers marry younger women. Boomers—those born between 1946 and 1964— are marrying and having children later. College bills are staring them in the face, their parents are old and may soon need a helping hand, and their job security is questionable.

If cosmetic surgery were a stock, it would have gone up several points after a recent *Wall Street Journal* column describing the dearth of jobs for older people, no matter how experienced and skilled they are. "Face it," warned the column, "no matter how secure you feel, you grow more vulnerable as you grow older." It advised "planning post-retirement careers by age forty-five," and staying up to date on matters big and small from computers to clothes. Some older people "aren't putting their best foot forward and it shows," carped one adviser to greybeards.

A week later, the *Journal*, citing a study by the National Bureau of Economic Research, reported that "pulchritude [pays] handsomely . . . ; the comely earn higher wages than the homely . . . ; good-looking people generate more money for their employers than their plain co-workers do"; and companies with more pretty people "generally had higher revenues." All these factoids are tossed into the blender when we're deliberating whether or not to have a surgical fix.

"In previous centuries," says anthropologist McCracken, "the individual was embedded in a family, social class, and ethnic group. You were somebody's son. You belonged to this community. People didn't feel themselves distinct. But today we have people getting progressively pushed out of their groups. You used to be able to count on being married for forty years and working for IBM for a certain number of years. Now, we have the sense of being less connected, and what connections we have can be severed more easily. We feel more distinct, separate, visible, vulnerable."

One IBM executive underwent cosmetic surgery to get a job promotion, reported a San Jose paper. Fearing the job would go to a younger person, forty-year-old "Jan," spent 10,000 dollars of her savings on a face-lift. Jan, of course, didn't tell her colleagues why she looked so good. But, P.S., she got the promotion.

Even Cindy Crawford—yes, the owner of the face so many women want to emulate—is feeling vulnerable now that she has turned thirty. "At my age," Cindy Crawford was quoted as saying recently, "you become more of a spokesperson." After a daily diet of confidence-threatening, bad-news bites, your wrinkles are one thing you don't want standing between you and job security.

Small wonder that between 1992 and 1994, a period marked by widespread corporate downsizing, there was a 50-percent increase in the number of patients undergoing wrinkle-diminishing chemical peels. Ageism and lookism may be illegal, but they are widely practiced. When qualifications are equal, the most attractive and vigorous-looking candidate often gets the job. Being old may be okay. But looking old is definitely not okay.

Like drugs targeted to receptor sites, cosmetic surgery advertisements target our insecurities:

"If the person you see in the mirror looks older than the person you feel like inside, we'd like to help you change that," says one seductive message. "For the young at heart who wish they had a face to go with it," beckons another. With that army of 76 million baby boomers heading over the hill, the only thing that could stop the multi-billion dollar cosmetic-surgery tsunami would be an anti-aging pill.

6:30 A.M.

It's my turn in the admitting office. My husband and I have been ushered into a cubicle furnished in Chippendale modular. After answering the basics, I'm asked by the admitting clerk, "Do you have a living will?" I do.

By now there is no turning back. I sign the consent forms, list my allergies to medications, the pills I'm taking, tell them whom to call in an emergency, pay in advance for the operating room and my two-night stay. (I've already pre-paid the otolaryngologist, the plastic surgeon, and the anesthesiology group.) The hospital accepts credit cards for its charges. *Ah, was it the face or the frequent flyer miles,* the ad would say.

I'm paying for this out of my own savings, as I did for my first face-lift. Although my husband J. has never tried to talk me out of surgery, his position is, "This is your caper," and refuses to contribute. I can say it's my body and my money, and if anything goes wrong, his conscience will be clear.

I am given my patient's bill of rights by a nurse/maitre d' and escorted down the poster-decorated hall to my semi-private room. Once again, J. shakes his head ever so slightly and gives me that "you're out of your mind" look which has become a staple of our mutually tolerant relationship. The countdown has begun.

I begin to wonder whether that trip to Phoenix had anything to do with my being here today.

Three

LOSING FACE

"I used to think cosmetic surgery was stupid. . . .
And now I don't."

—BIRTHDAY GREETING, DALE CARDS

A year before face-lift number two, when I had just started working on this book, "Libby," an old friend, sent an S.O.S. from Arizona, where she had settled. She was coming to New York, she said, and needed to talk to me, urgently. It wasn't hard to guess what was on her mind—she was approaching the mental roadblock called *fifty.*

Over lunch at Barney's, Libby pumped me for information about surgeons who were especially good at face-lifting. Had I heard of so-and-so in New York and what's his name in L.A.—you know, the one who did—and she names a well-known actress. The scoop was not for herself, but for a friend, she insisted, rather transparently. Personally, said Libby, she was looking forward to her "elderhood."

"But, if you're writing a book about this," she added, "you ought to come to Phoenix and talk to some women of the West. We're more athletic and body conscious than Easterners—and the plastic surgery there has accelerated."

When other business took me to Scottsdale, a Phoenix suburb, I took her up on the offer. Between Libby's contacts and mine, we put together a random sampling of fifteen women to talk nips and tucks.

I asked them to go around the table and introduce themselves. They were mostly working women, ranging in age from twenty-three to fifty-five, single and married, Caucasian and Hispanic. Though having had cosmetic surgery was not a condition of the invitation, two-thirds of my guests were no strangers to it. Looking back now on the snapshots I took that night, it's hard to tell who had had facial surgery and who hadn't.

I was the oldest in the group and when I owned up to my age, there was a burst of applause, proving just how deep-rooted age stereotypes are. I wasn't sure whether they were applauding because I was still working at sixty-seven or because I didn't fit their preconceived notion of that age.

Before making that trip to Scottsdale, I had wondered whether women of different generations could talk about this subject together. After my Southwestern sojourn, I wasn't wondering anymore. This topic transcends age, income, and lifestyle. Women, no matter what their age, are dismayed by what time does to the face. But they are deeply torn about taking surgical steps to restore their youthful appearance.

Depending on their age, women, as we know, take different measures to combat the effects of aging. There's a tacit agreement that any procedure performed without a knife is guilt-free (much in the way the dessert you didn't order, but only shared, is considered calorie-free). This may help explain why laser eye surgery is so popular. The laser can be used as a cutting instrument, but because it's presented as a relatively bloodless procedure, patients can pretend it doesn't count as surgery.

In plastic surgery as in sex, you don't lose your virginity till you go all the way—and taking that step is a moral decision my Arizona guests debated at length. They were less talkative about the factors that prompted their face work. It was as if it was so clearly necessary it didn't need to be explained. Some of what I heard was:

"I wasn't ready to look middle-aged. I wanted to look on the outside the way I felt on the inside."

"Am I happy looking at myself? I'm a terrible critic."

"I was in control. I was exercising. I lost weight. But I didn't feel I was together the way I wanted to be."

The unifying theme was one I've expressed myself: "Who's that woman in the mirror? I don't recognize her."

The face-lift is "about identity," says sociologist Kathy Davis. "For a woman who feels trapped in a body which does not fit her sense of who she is, cosmetic surgery becomes a way to renegotiate identity." The change from "my face" to "that other face" creeps up gradually. Misrepresentation is the leitmotif underscoring every before-and-after face-lift narrative. Just before she hit fifty, Cher, the would-be poster girl for plastic surgery, put it this way: "The idea of not being this way, of losing it all and somehow being less of a person just because I no longer look the same . . . that's kind of scary."

Sometimes there is an epiphany.

Washington gossip columnist Diana McLellan, in a memoir of her face-lift in *Washingtonian* magazine, told of how the seed was planted when she looked in the mirror and (appropriating Joan Rivers's jibe at Elizabeth Taylor) asked herself, "Who's that woman with more chins than the Hong Kong phone book?" The seed was nourished with bits of gossip and information, such as "Jackie O getting a facelift on her sixtieth birthday."

The Hypocritic Oath

Why is it that the only people who admire pleated faces are people who don't own them? It's fashionable to give lip service to older women. Fashion photographer Steven Meisel, explaining why he uses "older" models occasionally (by "older" he means Lisa Taylor at forty and Lauren Hutton at forty-six), said, "I think it is helpful for women to see mature images." At the young age of forty, Meisel himself boasted, privately, of having the lines in his face filled with various puffer-uppers. We can now forgive Dorothy Parker for her comment on her fiftieth birthday, "People ought to be . . . young or dead." She lived in a different era. But attitudes aren't all that different today. "I saw Angela Lansbury in an antique store the other day," jokes a comedian on late night TV. "They wanted eight hundred dollars for her."

"Bob Dole doesn't *have* ancestors," said Jay Leno. "You think of him as *being* an ancestor." Was it all those jokes about his age that prompted Dole to have a face-lift in 1997 in preparation, one assumes, for a shot at being First Husband?

And anyone who wants to be Camilla Parker Bowles—Prince Charles's lover, whom the tabloids have variously called, "that old boiler, old trout, old bag, prune, hatchet face, horse face ... weather-beaten, witch, vampire, frump"—please raise your hand. Death spared Diana, Princess of Wales, from such humiliations, observed columnist Liz Smith the day after Diana's death. "She died young and beautiful still. No one will ever write of Diana's 'middle-age' crisis or rush to print photos of the 'aging princess.' " But these jabs are nothing compared to Tanzania, Africa, where wrinkles and red eyes mark old women as mediums for witchcraft who must be abolished. "A son could kill his own mother simply because her eyes changed from normal to red."

The Bridges of Madison County was hailed as the romantic classic of the nineties—especially for middle-aged women, who are rarely the love interest in books and films. As one reader gushed, "It's not Tolstoy," but, "it will make you believe in love after the age of forty." And then came the disillusionment when we read in 1997 that the author, Robert James Waller, fifty-eight, had divorced his fifty-six-year-old wife Georgia and moved in with a thirty-four-year-old. Meanwhile, the craggy-faced Clint Eastwood, the director and co-star of the film adaptation of Bridges, in 1994 left his lover of six years and the mother of his child, the forty-plus actress Frances Fisher. In 1996, he married a newscaster less than half his age. So much for the promise of love after forty.

"We were once obliged to 'act our age,' " says anthropologist Grant McCracken in his book Plenitude. "Age instructions ... still shape the lives of ... millions," he says. "But everywhere we look we see little acts of refusal." For many, the face-lift is one such act, although others view it as a paradigm of conformity.

The face-lift is unique among plastic surgery procedures because it is designed to restore a physical condition, rather than serving as a vehicle for dramatic body-image adjustment.

Nonetheless, the decision to have one is not usually impulsive. The discourse of justification—can take months or even a few years. During that time, says Davis, the woman considering a lift builds her case for—or against—surgery, making comparisons of herself to others, debating the morality of the decision, defending it, and justifying it. "Taking action usually requires outside encouragement" from one or two people—rarely a spouse, who is usually opposed to any surgery. And the final step is reassurance.

Most people suffer a kind of myopia when it comes to their faces—at first they don't see the signs of aging. And if they do notice, they don't accept them. According to John and Marcia Goin (a plastic surgeon and psychologist, respectively), who have written extensively on the mind-set of the plastic surgery patient, "Body image does not age as rapidly as the physical body itself . . . [The] wrinkled and sagging facial and neck skin is never fully incorporated into the body image of aging individuals."

Who Me?

Regardless, time and again in the before-and-after narratives that have become staples of style pages and women's magazines, women talk about lengthy deliberations. In a *USA Today* story, Christine Royal, a Winston-Salem, NC woman, said that before she decided on a face-lift at forty, she spent two years "watching her face fall," and then started sleeping on her back hoping her loose jowls and saggy neck might straighten out.

Another long-term deliberator was Nienke Vandermeer, a former dancer, who admitted in *New York* magazine that she once thought plastic surgery was "narcissistic and frivolous, a foolish ploy to try to reverse time." That was before she developed a turkey gobbler neck. "I'd thought about it"—a face-lift—"for about a year and decided I was tired of camouflaging that shivering blob with high necks and long hair."

Because the means to the end is admittedly extreme—costly and risky—the person opting for surgery often insists the decision is out of character, said Davis. "I was always opposed to it," she'll say. "I'm not that type." "I never thought I was so vain."

That attitude was borne out at my nip-and-tuck discussion in Arizona. The propriety of tinkering with Mother Nature was on the table, right beside the finger sandwiches and the pasta salad. "CeCe," a thirty-one-year-old artist, was the first to raise the issue. "I feel trapped between vanity and less superficial values," she said. "I admire Asian cultures where the emphasis is on wisdom and education. I think it's sad we live in a culture in which so much emphasis is put on the appearance, materialism, and youth. But as long as that's the case," she reasoned, she had improved her contours with liposuction and ironed out deep-frown lines with a forehead lift.

"Ronnie," forty, a kitchen designer, said a fallen brow ran in her family and admitted to having had two brow- and eye-lifts—the first when she was thirty-one and again, recently. Although she's happy with the results, she said she feels like "a cheater."

"Maria," a physiotherapist, said from the age of ten she hated her broad, ethnic nose, but waited till her forties to attend to it. When none of her clients noticed the difference, Maria had an epiphany. "All these years I'd been worrying about my nose and I finally realized, you're not your hair, you're not your face, you're not your body—you are your internal soul." Still, she didn't want the old nose back.

"I think it's a shame that our society is so fixated on, you know, looks and material things, because it's really what's inside that counts," said "Georgia," a petite, fifty-four-year-old, pistol-packing rancher. "I don't see anything wrong with making improvements and maintaining." But, she said, she disapproves of it for young people "who don't appear to have anything physically wrong with them. They're looking for a fix, and you think, 'Where is this going? Where is the wisdom?' "

My pal Libby, a screen writer and a fitness buff, was another moralizer. It was clear from her body language (arms crossed) and the way she placed her chair (away from the table) that she was in a resistant mode. She told the group she had no qualms and no regrets about her nose job, done when she was in her teens ("It made my life better," she said), but she had serious misgivings about joining the face-lift club. "I'm worried about a culture that fears aging so much," said Libby, "we eventually sit around this table and no one looks old."

Thomas Rees, Manhattan's premier cosmetic surgeon before his recent retirement, urges compassion for those who utter the kind of righteous statements I heard in Arizona. "The people who tell you they want to grow old gracefully are concealing their true feelings about how they look," wrote Rees in his 1988 book *More Than Just A Pretty Face.* "The people who seem most negative are sometimes the most conflicted." That may explain why, so often, the women sounding off to me on the importance of aging naturally, turn around and confess that they've had their noses fixed or their eye bags removed and beg me not to reveal it.

"Trina," a fifty-one-year-old, divorced interior designer, was one person in my Arizona discussion group who arrived without qualms. When she was forty, she told the group, "I had a boob job and my nose done, at the same time. Six months ago, I had a brow lift, an upper and lower 'bleph' "—short for blepharoplasty, an eyelid lift—"a full face-lift, and my neck done. And I believe in it.

"I think anything we as women do to make ourselves feel better, we should do," Trina continued, adding that even the youngest of her relatives understood her feelings on the subject. It wasn't an issue of vanity. It was more the specter of aging. "My eight-year-old granddaughter is afraid I'll get old, and, to her, getting old means dying," said Trina. "I highly recommend surgery to any woman who really likes herself. It's not frightening and I didn't find it that painful. Discomfort is all I experienced," she said, "and some anxiety. My doctor made me stop smoking first and my anxiety from nicotine withdrawal was worse than my recovery."

As the evening wore on, Trina grew impatient with the moralizing of the other women. "I would just like to say something," she interjected. "We've been through the gamut here, mostly spiritual, about the way we look. And that's kind of foreign to me. I look at it as a design-construction-maintenance situation. This is my design. If it needs paint, I'll paint it; if it needs carpet, I'll carpet; if it needs a roof, I'll roof it. It's maintenance. I want my building to look as good as it can look for as long as it can. I want it to be vital, I want it to be alluring, I want to *feel* good in it. And my spirituality isn't mixed up with the way my building looks. Do it for yourself, because then you will feel good, and when you feel good about yourself you make other people feel good about themselves, and *then* they want to be with you."

Yes, No, Maybe

When it comes to plastic surgery, opined my friend "Nancy," a marketing executive, women can be divided into three categories: yes, no, and maybe. The Yeses "have a positive predisposition," said Nancy, who puts herself solidly in this category. "The Maybes don't look that bad yet. They're hoping to get away with a quick fix—liposuction under the chin or collagen shots." And the Nos? "They will never be interested," she said, taking them at their word.

Maybe I'm jaded, but I've stopped believing women's pronouncements on personal appearance issues. I've seen too many women, myself included, reverse themselves: "I'll never wear blue eyeshadow," they say, "I'll never tweeze my eyebrows," and the words most often eaten, "I'll never color my hair." Then one day, when the head is heavily salted, but light on the pepper, there is Ms. Principles, in the next chair in the salon with gook on her roots.

Those in the "No" category, feel the need to justify their decisions as much as the Yeses. In 1995, Penny Crone, the street-smart Fox television reporter in New York, who was forty-eight at the time, did an Emmy award-winning series on aging entitled "The Fountain of Youth." She kicked it off with the question "Who doesn't want to stay young?" She herself didn't want a face-lift and didn't think she needed one, but as a lark she let her viewers decide. "I'm putting my face in your hands," she announced. "If you think I look fabulous, vote No." And she was shocked by their response.

Thousands of votes poured in. "More people voted on my face-lift than on whether or not we should invade Bosnia," quips Crone. As the voting deadline neared, she says, the station's top brass worried that they would get stuck with the surgery bill. Crone was worried too, but not for financial reasons, she told me some time later over a cappuccino. The newscaster admitted that she doesn't relish getting older. She knows most of her colleagues will eventually have a nip or a tuck (if they haven't already, she says with a wink). But Crone doesn't want to go that route, partially because she believes some of her charm comes from a face that looks like it's been around the block more than once.

"I represent for women that you can keep going with the energy of a twenty-five-year-old and the personality of a sixteen-year-old," she told me in a voice that sounded like a rusty hinge. "Changing that would take away from what I stand for. When I get dressed in the morning, I see the lines in my face. When I'm out on assignment, I'll see twenty-five-year-old cops I'd like to jump in the sack with and they'll look at me like I'm their mother."

In the end, viewers voted down a facelift for Crone by a 4-percent margin, 52 to 48 percent. Crone had escaped the knife by the skin of her teeth. Or maybe by the skin of her skin.

Letty Cottin Pogrebin, pushing sixty, the Ms. Congeniality of the woman's movement, is pro-choice on artifice, but has taken a stand *against* a face-lift for herself—a position that may have more to do with personal phobias than political correctness. In voicing her misgivings, though, she speaks for many women.

In a lecture promoting her latest book *Getting Over Getting Older*, Pogrebin outlined her discourse of justification, describing how, at forty-nine, she "went into a tailspin . . . checking out wrinkles and crinkles and spreading waistlines." She described the angst of the aging woman "trapped in the wrong face with loose skin and deep lines," and feeling "misrepresented"—that word again. A suggestion by her dermatologist that she could look "a hundred percent better without those fat pouches under your eyes," inspired an inner debate on the politics of transformation.

Pogrebin thought of the friend who saved up three years for a 7,000-dollar neck lift and feels "born again"; then of another friend, who eventually turned out fine, but temporarily "suffered the torments of hell" after a face-lift, with "hideous swelling . . . corneas bruised . . . eyelids that wouldn't close." Or the chums who had no ill-effects but their faces look "strange, expressionless . . . almost unrecognizable"—a justifiable concern—"and nose jobs that left women looking almost the same as before" (which may have been the goal).

She acknowledged the importance of being beautiful, the possible job advancement, increased social contacts, improved self-esteem—not her problems, Pogrebin said, since she is self-employed, works at home, is married to man who likes her as she is, and isn't disfigured.

Isn't "bowing to the beauty standard" just "validating the idea that aging is something that has to be 'fixed' or 'cured'?" she wonders, although she concedes that every time she puts on blush or plucks her eyebrows she may be surrendering to unfair beauty standards.

What's really holding her back, however, are her own misgivings. The first: Her hemophobia—a life-long panic reaction at the sight of blood. Until she conquered it with therapy, she said, it was so severe, it used to send her to the hospital ten to fifteen times a year. The second is her belief—actually, a misconception—that you have to hide behind closed doors for six months waiting to heal—something she said she doesn't have time for. And neither do the 90,000 women currently undergoing face-lifts annually.

If Pogrebin had been at my dinner in Arizona, she could have met "Monica," a forty-nine-year-old insurance executive, who brought her before-and-after pictures to dinner. Ten days after her face-lift and chin implant, she said, "I went to a wedding."

The majority of patients, even those with high-visibility jobs like flight attendant—return to work and social life within one month. Bob Dole was a guest on Jay Leno's *Tonight Show* and on the Larry King show one month after his recent unacknowledged lift. Deep lifts that cause excessive swelling may require a two-month hideout, but that's rare. You may not see the *final* result for six months or a year, but that doesn't mean you have to stay behind closed doors for six months.

In spite of her reservations, said Pogrebin, she reserves the right to change her mind. Call her a "Maybe later."

Mixed Messages

Much of the negativity over body alteration reflects the long-standing religious and moral injunctions against any bodily corrections—even of congenital problems like a bulbous nose, cleft palate, or a port-wine stain on the cheek. Until the nineteenth century, anyone repairing birth defects was considered "meddling with the handiwork of God."

The grandfather of plastic surgery, Gaspare Tagliacozzi, the Bolognese anatomist who popularized the technique for rebuilding mutilated noses in the late sixteenth century, and wrote the first plastic surgery textbook, was condemned for his work while he was alive. And when he died, the church would not allow his remains to be buried in hallowed ground.

Today, body changes are an *ideological* offense and the chief of the body police is Naomi Wolf, who went from obscurity to celebrity by exposing all forms of vanity oppression in *The Beauty Myth*. In the chapter on "Violence," she blames greedy plastic surgeons for selling women a feeling of "terminal ugliness," and brands cosmetic surgery "beauty determinism"—as insidious as "women's invalidism," a nineteenth-century mechanism for controlling women's sexual impulses. Wolf advocates a sweeping cultural redefinition of beauty. "We don't need to change our bodies, we need to change the rules."

She shouldn't hold her breath.

"Naomi Wolf sees cosmetic surgery as vanity because she has the luxury of being young and beautiful," retorts sociologist Jacque Lynn Foltyn, author of the forthcoming book, *The Importance of Being Beautiful*. "But some older feminists, confronting their sagging jowls and drooping eyelids in the mirror, are doing a self-serving flipflop, excusing plastic surgery as feminine power."

Among the first was Gloria Steinem. In *Revolution From Within*, Steinem admits to a bias against any body change that isn't "necessary," but, as we saw before, she doesn't rule out changes that are "healthy and empowering"—such as her own eyelid operation that has enabled her to "get rid of those big glasses I'd been hiding behind for so long."

When Jane Bryant Quinn, the financial journalist and TV commentator, was considering facial surgery, she had to weigh the politics against the benefits. Her TV career "might well have ended by now if I hadn't [had a face-lift]," she told *Working Woman*. "As a card-carrying feminist, I wondered, 'Should I stand for the right to have wrinkles?' But then, I don't stand for the right to wear frumpy clothes. I finally decided I wasn't going to treat a face-lift as an ideological decision. The heck with it."

The idea of "natural" seems quaint, when we are implanting in our bodies everything from toe joints to artificial skin, vascular grafts and hybrid organs. We take vitamin supplements for pep, human growth hormone, melatonin, and antioxidants to beat the actuarial life-expectancy figures. We see better with eyeglasses, hear with cochlear implants, run faster with sneakers, keep our hearts beating with pacemakers, and achieve better erections with Viagra. But if the person whose advice you value doesn't believe in fooling with Mother Nature, you'll have a hard time walking into a cosmetic surgery operating room.

Sinful Feelings

Opposition from a family member is the only thing standing between "Susan," a fifty-three-year-old screenwriter, and her face-lift. Susan has lost patience with twice-yearly autologous fat injections (taken from her hips)—which she finds painful and expensive. "I used to subscribe to the idea that 'beauty is just skin deep' and 'it's what's inside that counts,' " she says, quite seriously. But that was before her jaw started sagging and she developed what she calls her chicken neck. "They're terribly aging," she says.

Susan's sister is violently opposed to surgery for Susan. "I agree with her, in principle," says Susan. "I resent the idea we must look young to be acceptable to men. It would be nice to weigh three hundred pounds and be accepted." But Susan has her own justification. "This is the real world," she says. "People judge you by your looks. My sister is thirteen years younger than I am. She hasn't crossed that [appearance] border yet."

For aeons, even before Tagliacozzi's run-in with the church, women have been shamed, blamed, warned, and mocked about their vanity. Damnation was the punishment for going to God with a face that wasn't one's own. In the beginning, cosmetics, hair dyes, and dangerous skin treatments were the forbidden fruits. But by the twentieth century, plastic surgery had become the offender. The early cosmetic surgeons weren't even the social equivalent of today's used-car salesmen. So-called reputable doctors did their best to discourage women from patronizing "quacks." In view of the bad press cosmetic surgery attracted, *Ladies Home Journal* showed guts by publishing "Why Grow Old?"—probably the first plastic-surgery shopping story—in 1922.

The writer Ethel Lloyd Patterson approached the subject with fear and fascination—she was, she thought, the ideal age, thirty-nine. The paternalistic physicians she interviewed branded "cosmo-plastique-surgery" frivolous, dangerous, and immoral. "A woman of forty or more," one general surgeon told her, "ought to be ashamed to have a face without a wrinkle." Women who would undergo this surgery, he said condescendingly, were "doll women." Surgeons who would perform such work might leave a woman disfigured for life.

A skin specialist quoted in the article blamed women for their falling faces. He said he had "no sympathy" for the vanity problems of "ladies of leisure. . . . If a woman with your chances in life today does not remain young indefinitely it is because she has sold her birthright for a mess of pottage, smoking, drinking, eating too much or indulging in physical irregularities." His cure-all for aging was pure oxygen. "Tell them," he said, "to exercise every morning in front of an open window for ten minutes."

Face-lifting was probably crude in those days; there were good reasons to fear it. Describing the result of a lift undergone by one fiftyish woman, the reporter wrote: "Her unnatural smoothness of contour . . . made my flesh creep."

Still, despite the scoldings, the warnings, and the risks—and remember, at that time the anesthesia was local—topical or injected cocaine—Patterson was intrigued. She said she could imagine herself succumbing to the surgical fix. If she had "sorry and discontented lines . . . from nose to mouth" and if her personal doctor would recommend a good surgeon, she concluded, she would consider having a cheek lift (what we would call a mini-lift or a skin-lift, today).

If you can't actually ban an activity, or damn people for doing it, a time-honored behavior-modification tactic is to mock it into being socially unacceptable. Osbert Sitwell drew blood in his 1930 short story "Charles and Charlemagne," about London's Lady de Montfort, whom he described as a "pioneer of the Peter Pan movement," a breed who find "something glorious in never growing up" . . . and "wish to remain young out of season."

More recently, one of the most merciless put-downs was a 1995 *Elle* editorial, "Very Plastic Surgery: What Are We Doing to Ourselves?" The copy was cruel. "They look like aliens, these women, with their big unblinking eyes, their doll noses and tiny chins, that eerie, poreless, rubberized sheen on their skin. . . . These women seem kind of tragic to me . . . so girlishly eager to please they'll cut off offending parts of themselves." One of New York's alternative publications imagined a Disneyland type attraction, where people drink "collagen cola" as they stroll on "Cosmetic Alteration Boulevard." But ridiculing Tammy Faye Bakker's over-the-top mascara hasn't killed mascara sales.

"Aging is difficult for everyone," observes Thomas Rees. "Anyone who tells you otherwise is masking a fear, or mouthing clichés." As the birthdays roll around, one by one, people who once voted No to facial surgery, begin to say Maybe. It took a cancer scare for author Meg Cox, a former *Wall Street Journal* reporter, to acknowledge her investment in her face. Ten years earlier, she had turned down a modeling contract to finish college. Two years ago when she turned forty-two, a tiny blemish at the tip of her photogenic nose was diagnosed as malignant. The cancer was successfully removed but she was astounded at how disturbed she was by the minuscule indentation of her nose she was left with. "I used to think I wasn't vain. After all, I had walked away from modeling. But you can't live in this culture without being concerned about how you look. You want to make the most of your best features. That's why the cancer hit me hard. I realized, I'm over forty. In demographers' eyes, I am middle-aged. I don't look my age and never did and I've always felt a bit smug, thinking it would always be like that. But suddenly you see it"— aging—"is going to happen to you and it's very sobering."

Cox had her first child when she was forty-one. Now she worries about how she'll look when it's time to take her toddler to school. Adding another supporting argument to her dossier, she says, "I don't want him to think he has an old mommy."

Votes of Confidence

After the case is built and justified, it often takes a catalyst to get you to set a date—a major event—like a family wedding, a class reunion, a public appearance (book tour, award ceremony, or a court date).

Encouragement plays a role, too. It used to come from one or two good friends. It still does. But it can also come from a brave-new-world media story about a miracle laser, or an inspirational before-and-after story like Diana McLellan's *Washingtonian* report on her own face-lift. The issue it ran in was the magazine's all-time best-seller. Seven years later, says McLellan, "I still get several telephone calls a month from total strangers all over the country asking my advice. They want to know, Am I pleased? Would I do it again? They need encouragement."

Nothing is as influential as encouragement from an admired friend who has been there. In the middle of my own deliberations about my first face-lift, I got a call from my former literary agent, now deceased, a grand dame and a beauty many years my senior—how many, I never asked. I tell her I'm thinking of having a face-lift and I'm terribly conflicted. She exclaims, "That's marvelous! Do it! This is your outer skin; it needs a nip and a tuck. So what? There's no vanity in that. You're like me. You have no age."

"Maybe I should grow old gracefully," I say.

"I don't want to grow old gracefully, and I don't accept it," she says emphatically. "I never fussed with my appearance. But I would pass a mirror and say, 'Who is that? It looks like my mother.' I had surgery when I was sixty-five. It made my life better."

Without support, the guilt and shame can torpedo the endeavor. That was the case with Nonnie, a social Brahmin in one of America's most affluent zip codes. Now that her kids are grown, Nonnie devotes herself almost full-time to worthy causes—the homeless, literacy, AIDS, the local symphony orchestra. She never thought of herself as a person who would obsess about a few wrinkles, even a few dozen wrinkles. To her, authenticity—in antiques, in a string of pearls, and in faces—is a virtue.

That's why Nonnie was so perplexed by her secret obsession. At fifty-three, she desperately wanted an eye lift. "I was the last person in the world you'd expect to do this," she says. "I was enjoying aging naturally. I didn't mind my gray hairs and wasn't planning to do anything about them." But something was happening to her eyes. "My younger sister and I both inherited the same droopy lids. My sister had it taken care

38

LIFT

of and was pleased with the result. I thought it was the wrong thing for *me* to do. It just seemed so . . . *self-indulgent.*

Nonnie could be the textbook case described by Robert M. Goldwyn, a Harvard plastic-surgery professor, in his book *The Patient and Plastic Surgery.* "[She] may feel ashamed about having cosmetic surgery and usually does. . . . Friends may consider her foolish; her husband may call her 'crazy'; and her family doctor may be strongly opposed." For Nonnie, the venture—from deliberation to justification to action—was, as one of Goldwyn's patient's described it, "a lonely vigil."

Oddly, to find a surgeon, Nonnie, who wouldn't dream of buying curtains from an ad in the Yellow Pages, opened the phone book. "I don't know what got into me," she says. "It was so unlike me. I selected three doctors from their ads and interviewed them. I chose one, a woman. I could easily have asked for references, but I didn't. I just wanted to do it and get it over with." Even after setting the date, Nonnie told no one— "not my husband, my children, my sister, my family doctor." Most cosmetic surgeons refuse to operate on patients who are excessively secretive about their surgery or whose spouse says no.

The weekend before her surgery date, Nonnie began having serious second thoughts. "My daughter announced she was pregnant and I thought, She could use that twenty-five hundred dollars I was spending. I was terribly conflicted. Still, I was determined," says Nonnie. She arranged for a neighbor to pick her up afterward. "We often help one another out. I confided in him. He thought it was a great idea." That was the only encouragement Nonnie had, and it wasn't enough.

On the appointed day she got as far as the operating table. The I.V. was inserted in her arm. "The minute the sedative hit my body," she recalls, "I had an overwhelming sense of anxiety. I started shaking. 'Stop this!' " I cried out. " 'I can't go through with this! I feel horrible.' Suddenly, I knew what I was doing was wrong, *terribly wrong.*"

The anesthetist removed the I.V. A nurse helped Nonnie into a chair. "The surgeon was terribly annoyed," says Nonnie. " 'This is highly irrational,' the surgeon told me."

Nonnie isn't sure whether it was the overwhelming guilt, lack of trust in the doctor, a reaction to the narcotic, or a combination. Whatever precipitated the anxiety attack, it unleashed a flood of repressed emotions that led to a reevaluation of her marriage and her life. "Maybe the crisis would have happened anyway," she says. "I don't know. It was like a nervous breakdown. I'm still working it through."

In spite of the trauma, Nonnie hasn't stopped wanting surgery. "I hope when I get my life straightened out, I'll get my eyes done. I still want to do it." (Two years later, after therapy, a separation from her husband, and finding a supportive surgeon who came highly recommended, Nonnie did finally get her eye-lift—under local anesthesia—and couldn't be happier. "I don't look sixteen, I look my age, but there are no more bags," she says.)

Don't Ask, Don't Tell

Celebrities and politicos may have the weakest support system—because they need to be so secretive. Even their best friends don't know if and when they've had surgery. "It's the one question I'm not allowed to ask her," says the personal publicist of a major Hollywood star.

One legend invited me to her pied-à-terre to talk about face-lifts. She needed a sounding board for her "discourse of justification" and trusted I wouldn't reveal her identity. "It's a private thing," she said. "There's a disadvantage in others knowing." She didn't relish the idea of being outed in gossip columns or becoming the butt of jokes on late-night talk shows. Surrounded by biographical mementoes—a satin slipper, in which she danced at the height of her fame, and portraits of her at various stages in her career—the transient nature of beauty was palpable. Now in her early sixties, she is still being offered parts—albeit older ones. She assured me she has no desire to turn back the clock to the days when she was a ravishing newcomer; she just wants to look as good as she can for as long as she can.

She talked about the commitment it takes to remain glamorous. "Millions of people loved Dietrich's face," said the star. "If she hadn't had face-lifts she wouldn't have been the glamorous persona she created. These are choices stars make to live up to the success and adoration. It does not just happen. One has to make an effort—manicures, pedicures, this and that. It's a huge job."

"I was first aware that I was aging when I reached thirty-four," she said. "I saw these little lines when I looked in the mirror. Oh God, I said to myself, it's happened. I had never heard of anyone going for surgery that young. Perhaps one day, I thought." It wasn't until four or five years ago, she says, she was aware of losing face. "I thought I should do something. I noticed these things . . . it was something about my eyes. Are they more sunken because I'm older? And I have two vertical lines between the eyebrows that I don't want. So I'm thinking, Can anything be done or is it better to just let it go? This is the dilemma."

After the self-scrutiny comes the justification. "In the theater, the only people who can see you are in the first three rows," she says. "But in films, the screen is so big. I know a few actresses who have had their faces lifted. Suddenly you realize there are no crow's-feet. They look magnificent, not younger. Fresher. That is what one aims for. You're just dealing with what God gave you. Why not? God won't mind."

Show business is so competitive, it's said, one star's rejuvenation often drives her competitors to take similar measures. But a Yes vote from a prominent woman affects more than her own circle. If the news leaks out, or if some columnist makes a smart guess, the rest of us have one more influential role model. Just as we slavishly imitated Joan Crawford's power shoulders and Veronica Lake's bedroom hair, now we follow the leaders to the operating room.

Probably no single group has done more to set the standards of beauty—and then conform to them with surgery—than movie stars, although their publicity machinery would have us believe their appearance is all natural. But we're not visually challenged. We can see how they've changed—or in some cases, stayed the same for an unusually long time.

As Robin Leach quipped in the BBC documentary, *Hollywood Women*, the initials "L.A. stand for liposuction and augmentation." And nothing can stop the vast makeover machine. Even an earthquake of 6.6 on the Richter scale could not close down the operating rooms for long. Los Angeles rumbled to a standstill at 4 A.M. on Monday, January 17, 1994.

Later that morning, at plastic surgeons' offices throughout the area—roadblocks, collapsed freeways, and aftershocks notwithstanding—many patients scheduled for elective surgery showed up.

"We had patients waiting outside our door on Monday morning," said an assistant to Steven Hoefflin, the controversial plastic surgeon, who is known for performing many operations on Michael Jackson's nose. He was in the operating room using backup generators within forty-eight hours.

Cosmetic surgery and the entertainment industry have been co-dependent since they were both in their infancy. Hollywood has for nearly a century been turning the barely dumpy into the exceedingly dishy with diet, electrolysis, teeth-capping, chemical peels, and, yes, plastic surgery. "The studios ran their lives," says Richard Aronsohn, a veteran cosmetic surgeon in Los Angeles. "The stars did what they were told or else they didn't act." Louis B. Mayer, for instance, advised the budding Greta Garbo to get her teeth fixed and to lose weight because Americans didn't like their movie stars fat.

A defining moment in the history of cosmetic surgery—and its relation to films—was the invention of the film close-up around 1908 (not long after the first face-lift), by director D. W. Griffith and cameraman G. W. "Billy" Bitzer. "The close-up made ... performers into stars," wrote British cultural critic Clive James, in his book *Fame in the Twentieth Century*. It changed the relationship "between those [being] looked at and those doing the looking. . . . It was a way for the human race to worship itself in ideal form." Makeup, lighting, special lenses, and lens coatings—such as Vaseline and gauze—can correct only so much. Gloria Swanson once said, "We didn't need dialogue, we had faces." Of course, to preserve hers, she underwent seven face-lifts in her sixty-year career.

The first superstar to undergo facial rejuvenation surgery was the French thespian Sarah Bernhardt—the greatest star of her day. Bernhardt was born in 1844, and, according to one biographer, she never lied about her age, but "clung stubbornly to the self-delusion that in appearance she was younger than most of her associates." Still seductive in her sixties, she chose a young Adonis—one of Rodin's models—for her leading man and her lover. But even Bernhardt couldn't stop the clock.

When she began to age visibly, and the characters she played didn't, the critics turned against her.

The details are sketchy, but apparently Bernhardt's first face-lift was performed in the U.S. in 1912, when she was sixty-eight (just before the filming of *Queen Elizabeth*, her movie debut). When Bernhardt returned to France, after a triumphal American tour, recalled French cosmetic surgeon Suzanne Noël in her memoirs, "all the newspapers remarked that, by means of a practical operation performed on the scalp, [the actress] had regained a surprising degree of youthfulness." Not a bad reference for a fledgling procedure.

Fanny Brice, the Ziegfeld Follies' "Funny Girl," was the next major star to make plastic surgery news. Her nose surgery in August 1923, when she was thirty-one, generated so much hoopla, said the *Times*, "One might think it the greatest engineering feat since the building of the Panama Canal." Criticizing her for trying to hide her ethnicity, Dorothy Parker wrote that Brice "cut off her nose to spite her race." Interestingly, Parker (nee Rothschild) was half Jewish and was deeply ambivalent about her own Jewishness. Years after she became Mrs. Edwin Pond Parker II, she told friends she "had wanted to marry Eddie because he had a nice, clean name." But Brice, who never hid her origins—after all, she got her start in Yiddish theater—insisted she just wanted to look prettier so she could play more dramatic roles, especially Nora in *The Doll's House*.

Brice wanted her conspicuous nose made more normal. "I am tired of having to fit my hats to the curve of my nose rather than the needs of my temperament." she said. "No woman on the stage of today can afford to have a nose that is likely to keep on growing until she can swallow it."

"Other artists," observed an approving editorialist in the *Times*, "would accept the limitation and go on doing comedy; Miss Brice boldly decides to abolish the inhibitory nose." (Coincidentally, the other cause célèbre in the paper that week was the case of the couple in Massachusetts who were granted the right to change their name from Kabotchnik to Cabot, over the objections of the Cabot family, who felt the distinguished name would give the Kabotchniks an undeserved advantage, the same advantage many people silently resent when people like Brice appropriate a nondenominational nose.)

But Brice's surgery wasn't successful on any level. The difference from the old Fanny wasn't sufficient to make her conventionally pretty—but just enough to make her less funny. And in a particularly bitter twist, the new nose was blamed for her subsequent divorce from Nicky Arnstein—the first instance where plastic surgery was " 'responsible for alienating the affections of a husband.' " The divorce papers filed by Brice's lawyer claimed that after the surgery, Arnstein (incomprehensibly) " 'found her so much more beautiful, he was uncomfortable in her presence and' began 'seeking the society of other . . . plainer women.' "

It wasn't long before cosmetic surgery was a thriving, but hush-hush specialty in movieland. In the early years, surgery mostly involved noses, eyes, and ears. "Noses cost fifty dollars and usually an actor was referred by an agent who got a twenty-five-dollar kickback," said Edward Lamont, one of the town's early plastic surgeons. After Rudolf Valentino's death in 1926, his older brother Albert Guglielmi tried to recreate himself in Valentino's image. After seven nose jobs, "he still lacked 'a nose that the camera will like.' " In the late forties, producer Joe Schenk advised an aspiring movie actor named Marlon Brando to get his nose straightened if he wanted to get ahead. Brando refused. The bump on his nose was the result of a fall, and he thought it gave his face character. But he was in the minority. Eventually Nanette Fabray, Carmen Miranda, Peggy Lee, Marlo Thomas, and dozens of other male and female stars would have their noses done—some, like Miranda, with less than felicitous results.

"*Most* celebrities . . . have had something done," writes Michael Merron, a Hollywood makeup artist in his recent book *Makeover Miracles*. Even great talents and beauties. When she was starting out in films, Marlene Dietrich had her upper rear molars removed to achieve a sunken cheek look. On their way *up*, stars like Hedy Lamarr (touted as the most beautiful woman in the world) and Merle Oberon had surgery to photograph *better*. And on their way *down*, Joan Crawford, Lana Turner, Burt Lancaster, Robert Mitchum, John Wayne—and Hedy Lamarr—had work done so they would photograph *younger*.

Lamarr, June Havoc, and Milton Berle were featured in a 1948 *Look* magazine piece on nose surgery. "Though conservatives may look askance," said the text by Geri Trotta, "theater people, with their usual avant-garde acceptance of the new, have done an invaluable service in taking the hush-hush out of plastic surgery." Berle, who was just beginning a wildly successful career in television, was so delighted with this new profile, wrote Trotta, he had given "beak" jobs as Christmas gifts to friends and associates.

Yes, Even Marilyn

In 1949, Marilyn Monroe was a seventy-five-dollar-a-week contract player who was "getting nowhere fast." After overhearing someone at a party refer to her as "a chinless wonder," Monroe consulted plastic surgeon John Pangman who diagnosed "a mild flatness of the chin" and performed a cartilage graft. A few days after the operation, Monroe was called to test for a bit part. She put off the audition for a week, explaining that she had fallen on her chin. When she finally took the test, the director told her, " 'Honey, you should have cut your chin two years ago.' " She got the part, and the film, believed to be *The Asphalt Jungle*, released in 1950, would be the turning point in Monroe's career.

About the same time, it is said plastic surgeon Michael Gurdin, removed "a slight bump of cartilage from the tip of [Monroe's] nose." Monroe returned to Gurdin in 1962 after she fell (or some believe, was beaten up by her boyfriend). She was concerned, mistakenly, that her nose was broken.

Monroe's 1962 nose x-rays are kept, today, under lock and key in another Beverly Hills office. These relics—in their folder marked with an assumed name—exert a strange fascination, like the tooth of the Buddha. The goddess knew that her fame depended on maintaining her appearance. "Nothing alienates an audience from a star—especially a female star—more than her aging," wrote Jib Fowles, invoking a quote from Monroe, who said, "When my looks start to go, so will most of my fans."

All too often, stars, in an attempt to buy time, were willing guinea pigs for every new and questionable technique from deep phenol skin peels (Mae Murray) to liquid-silicone breast injections. It is believed that

Pangman—who was one of the pioneers of breast implants, well before the silicone-gel era—implanted Ivalon-sponge in Monroe's breasts in the fifties. She may also have had liquid-silicone injections in her breasts. Shortly before Monroe's death in 1962, "her breasts were infected," says Rosemary Eckersley, widow of plastic surgeon Franklin Ashley. "Marilyn wanted Frank to do something about them, but he wouldn't." More accurately, he couldn't. It's almost impossible to remove free silicone after it's injected.

Plastic surgery got an immense boost in the 1950s from Cinemascope and television, which magnified every pore. Before the advent of these technologies, a face-lift was considered a last resort. If an actress's face was looking wrinkled, prior to starting a film, she would have a rejuvenating skin peel or an electric facial—anything to avoid or postpone having a lift. Photography, lighting, and makeup tricks could take years off an actress's face—even wash out the severe acne Merle Oberon suffered from reactions to makeup. Lighting technicians would spend hours preparing for her scenes, using a plaster cast of her head as a stand-in.

For stars with loose skin there was the "Hollywood Lift"—a special contraption made of glue, silk thread, and rubber bands. Makeup artists used it to pull up many a sagging face. But the tugging was hard on the ears and the rubberbands would sometimes snap in the middle of a scene. But the advent of larger screens and better film clarity eventually made surgical nips and tucks unavoidable. "A tight closeup magnifies the face hundreds of times. The smallest mole shows up," said Westmore. "In the old days we used heavy makeup base, today we're using thinner makeup and you can see the texture and coloring of the face."

Television, which had greater magnification but smaller lighting budgets, sent actors to cosmetic surgeons in droves. Suddenly, male actors "discovered facial folds, bags under their eyes, baldness, ears sticking out, traumatic scars, a crooked nose" and wanted them fixed, recalled Michael Gurdin. Some Hollywood denizens approached surgery flamboyantly. The story may be apocryphal, but it's said that in order to choose a nose surgeon, one high-placed Hollywood wife, who wanted a very conservative operation, gave a luncheon for a dozen friends—each of whom had had a nose job—and compared the results.

Woolworth heiress Barbara Hutton—related to Hollywood by her brief marriage to Cary Grant—is said to have traveled with her own anesthesiologist and recuperated from her face-lift at the Bel Air hotel wearing a different color sari and matching jewels every day—a red sari with rubies, a green one with emeralds, and a blue one with sapphires. Lucille Ball wanted to enter the hospital, incognito, for an eye-lift, so she cooked up a caper worthy of an *I Love Lucy* episode, says one of her closest friends who was part of the scenario. " 'We'll go at night,' " Ball told the friend, " 'We'll dress like cleaning ladies; we'll carry mops. No one will recognize me.' Of course, everyone did," recalls the accomplice. Jolie Gabor—mother of Zsa Zsa and Eva—on the other hand, wanted to tell the world. She introduced her surgeon at a coming-out party for her face-lift in Palm Springs.

Most film folk pretended, however, never to have had surgery and snubbed their surgeons socially. Gurdin, who, it is rumored, pinned back Clark Gable's ears and revised Elizabeth Taylor's tracheotomy scar, was barely acknowledged at social events. "People would freeze when they saw Michael," recalls his widow. "He had operated on most of the people in the room. But he never could acknowledge it in any fashion."

Having surgery out of town was one way to avoid detection. Joan Crawford and Gary Cooper went to John Converse in New York for face-lifts. (After Cooper's death in 1961, Cooper's widow married Converse.) Sources say Bette Davis, who denied ever having work, went to New York's Tom Rees, a young member of Converse's staff, for a face-lift. To explain their improved looks, actors credited a special diet, sheep-cell injections in Switzerland, a new facialist.

The Beginning of the End of Guilt

The face-lift finally "came out" in the sixties, along with the women's liberation movement, the birth control pill, and the social reconstruction of middle age. People didn't feel they had to drop out anymore when they reached a certain age. Aging was becoming more flexible, and cosmetic surgery removed some of the stigmata of aging while making extended middle age more credible.

Harper's Bazaar gave the lift its seal of approval in its June 1960 report that began: "The Wish to Be Beautiful is part of every woman." Writer Geri Trotta acknowledged that looking young was as much a matter of economics as of vanity and that cosmetic surgery had moved beyond "the unwholesome hush of conspiracy, the aura of guilty secrecy. . . . Despite having been the object of derision, misinformation and almost superstitious ignorance, the face lift [it was then spelled without a hyphen], in the past decade, has become perhaps the second most popular cosmetic operation. . . . Age is the universal adversary and its milestones can be less than lovely." The operation, Trotta explained, took four to five hours and required a hospital stay of several days. As for secrecy, said Trotta, "No woman is willing to advertise her face-lift, but . . . she might larkily admit it to her friends as she might mention dyeing her hair."

The mainstreaming of cosmetic surgery had begun. A year later *McCall's* debunked several myths about face-lifting, especially the one that purports most face-lifts are "performed on vain, rich, idle women."

If there was any doubt, the following year, the *Ladies Home Journal* published "The Diary of a Face Lift." The author was an anonymous housewife who said she saved from her food allowance and took odd jobs to pay for the operation. She leveled with readers about the discomforts (fluid accumulated in the neck that had to be drained; itching scalp, nearly intolerable on thirteenth day) and the triumph—when she returned home, after a six-week recuperation out of town, her best friend said, "Oh, I hate you."

Little by little, women were being educated about the wonders of the face-lift and relieved of their guilt for wanting one. By 1964, *McCall's* reported that the face-lift is "the most common of facial operations." But, as unlikely as it may seem, nothing did more for face-lift acceptance than a wigged-out, self-denigrating comedienne named Phyllis Diller, whose career was built on wisecracks about her "spectacular lack of success at the beauty parlor."

In 1971, just months before Gloria Steinem, in the debut January 1972 issue of *Ms.*, urged women to "seize control of your life," Diller underwent a face-lift and proceeded to blab about it—in her act, on talk shows, and later in her first-person account in *Pageant* magazine, "What Every Woman Should Know About My Face-lift."

Diller risked "alienating the not-so-glamorous housewives" who were her audience, but her timing was right. It was the dawn of the age of talk-show confessionals and the public was ready for straight talk from celebrities. When Diller admitted it was no laughing matter to face the world with wrinkles and jowls and a crooked smile, ordinary women empathized. They hung on her descriptions of the incisions, the gory details of recovery—"looking like you've been hit by a car at fifty miles an hour"—the post-op fatigue, the stitch removal, and the thrill after a month when she first put on eye makeup and found there were no crows feet, sagging chin, or crooked nose.

"I can't begin to tell you how wonderful I feel," she enthused. "I'm a new woman! All my life, I had this complex about my nose. That's gone now. I feel like a million, as though someone gave me back twenty years of my life!" Since Diller didn't have a so-called "ethnic" nose, no one accused her of denying her roots and no apologies were necessary.

A nerve was touched. All over America, women said to themselves, "I could do that." The mail poured in. She still gets it. " 'Will it hurt?' 'How long will it last?' and 'How much will it cost?'—in that order," says Diller, ticking off the most frequently asked questions. "I assure them there is no pain, it will last five to ten years, and the cost depends on many things."

Diller subsequently underwent other procedures (teeth bonding, tat-tooed eyeliner, a brow lift, cheek implants, chemical peel, and liposuc-tion) and became a one-woman education program, supplying anyone who asked with a chronological list of her renovations and the doctors who performed them.

The surgeon who did Diller's first face-lift, Franklin Ashley, had treated stars with bigger names. He rebuilt Ann-Margret's face when she fell twenty-two feet from a stage platform in a Lake Tahoe nightclub in 1972. He did a face-lift on Fred Astaire and an eye-lift on John Wayne. Ashley was a big-game hunter, and one animal-activist star reportedly bolted out of his office after seeing his elephant-foot stool. But, no matter how many luminaries Ashley treated, he considered Diller his landmark.

Because of Diller's forthrightness, says one L.A. surgeon, "the public's attitude about cosmetic surgery went, in one decade, from fear to accep-tance to desire."

Today, in some circles, you almost have to apologize for *not* having surgery. The 1980s and 1990s have seen an explosion of cosmetic-surgery reportage. There's been more media coverage of cosmetic surgery in the last seven *years* than in the preceding seven *decades*. One thing remains constant: Practically the only people willing to talk about the subject are comedians. Where once gabbed Fanny Brice, Milton Berle, Jackie Gleason (who went public about his face-lift in *People* in 1977), and Phyllis Diller—we have Carol Burnett, Roseanne, and Joan Rivers, and a handful of straighter people willing to make fun of themselves— Mary Tyler Moore, Dolly Parton, and Cher.

Included in the credits on a 1983 comedy album, Rivers thanked Dr. Frank Kamer the plastic surgeon who did her first face-lift. "I came out," she said, "because it's so mean, so cruel, so unfair when all these famous women tell you it's just good health that makes them look like this. . . . You take your car to be Simonized. You get your clothes cleaned. Why not a little job under your chin?"

Anyone curious about Dolly Parton's pick-me-ups and the names of the doctors who performed them can buy her autobiography, *Dolly: My Life and Other Unfinished Business*. She admits to having had "nips and tucks and trims and sucks, boobs and waist and butt and such, eyes and chin and back again, peels and pills and other frills."

Not everyone wants to emulate Roseanne, but her face-lift was a convincing ad for its positive affects. Roseanne also taught the public the "self-esteem" justification. Putting a nineties spin on her four-year beautification project (face-lift, nose job, breast reduction, liposuction, and tummy tuck), Roseanne confessed she changed her nose because it reminded her of her father, whom she has accused of sexually abusing her. Surgery, she said, "was part of my physical recovery."

But among young dramatic stars, the cosmetic-surgery backlash is significant. Recent Academy-Award nominee Elisabeth Shue, for example, said she'd sooner switch careers than "have lots of cosmetic surgery." But moral positions can shift, as Jessica Lange confirmed. "Five years ago, I would have said no way," Lange told one columnist in 1994. "But as you age, you start thinking, well, there's always that option."

One Hollywood plastic surgeon has learned to be skeptical of naysayers. "It is very common for young actresses to proclaim they'll never have plastic surgery—as if they'll never get old," says John Williams, who was briefly married to Eva Gabor and has operated on scores of famous faces. "But, almost invariably, when they do begin to age, they change their minds, often becoming obsessed with what we can do."

Secrets and Lies

When celebrities do change their minds, secrecy is essential. To maintain patient privacy, another Hollywood plastic surgeon, who had a star-studded clientele, kept a list of monikers (often his nurses' names) to assign to famous patients. Artificiality "precipitates negativity," says Jib Fowles. It "destroys the star's intrinsic worth."

The secrecy can become obsessive and the denials just plain ludicrous. "I had Zsa Zsa Gabor in my office one day," says one L.A. surgeon. "I could see the scars from across the room, and she told me, 'I've never had anything done.' "

Even bi-monthly collagen shots can be devaluing, explains an up-and-coming Hollywood actress, I'll call "Brenda." No one ever spelled out the rules for her but she understands them. "Natural beauty is valued more than manufactured beauty. Having too much surgery makes a person seem insecure." And no matter how much effort one puts into one's appearance, "no one wants to look like she's trying too hard."

No one would know, if it weren't for the tabloids that pay for tips. "There is always someone pushing the wheelchair, who can't resist telling," says Janet Charlton, a *Star* columnist. Meanwhile, the stalkerazzi trail the stars to their cosmetic surgeons' offices. (When Lisa Marie Presley, newly wed to Michael Jackson, checked in to a private clinic on a Saturday for some work—the nature of which has never been disclosed—there was "a photographer behind every bush," said her surgeon, Edward Terino.)

Celebrity biographies used to include every secret *except* the subject's cosmetic surgery. But more and more, nothing is glossed over. Suzy

Menkes' 1987 biography of the Duchess of Windsor reveals she had at least three face-lifts: two in London and the last one in Paris. "She wasn't so much frightened of getting old," said her friend, Jacqueline de Ribes. "It was an aesthetic thing." Though not everyone's aesthetic. By 1971, said Cecil Beaton, the Duchess's "face was so pulled up that the mouth stretched from ear to ear."

The recent Sally Bedell Smith biography of Pamela Harriman gives a slice-and-stitch description of her face-lift, even mentioning the doctor's name. And in the book *The Devil's Candy*, the saga of the making of the film *Bonfire of the Vanities*, author Julie Salamon reports that Melanie Griffith, one of the stars, apparently had breast implants during filming.

Cher isn't waiting for her biographer. She is the Gypsy Rose Lee of plastic-surgery exposure, teasing that, "I am the equivalent of a counterfeit twenty-dollar bill," while covering herself with a press release admitting to nothing more than rhinoplasty and breast surgery. Anyone who alleges Cher has undergone more surgically—like having ribs removed to get a smaller waist (an operation no reputable doctor would perform) or cheek implants (both of which the entertainer has denied, emphatically)—risks a lawsuit. Cher's periodic disappearances and reappearances with a new look, the ensuing conjecture by the media, followed by denials or limited disclosures aren't preparations for a new performance, they are the performance—her act, so to speak. Her transformations, however they are accomplished, says Jib Fowles, "add a texture to Cher that others don't have. That's part of her great talent. She sacrifices herself for us."

But while the exposures titillate, they also inspire. We may be disillusioned to find that the physical characteristics we seem to envy (one actress's cheekbones, another's pouty lips, or still another's newly taut neck) may owe more to plastic surgery or to Botox injections than to Mother Nature; it was a blow to find that Jane Fonda's sharp jawline and beautiful body weren't entirely the result of her workouts. In various interviews, she admitted to face and body work. But we got over it. She asked for understanding—and many of her fans showed their support by following her into the operating room. While revelations of surgical artifice have made us more skeptical of stars' authenticity—their claims to fame—as Joshua Gamson pointed out in his study of celebrity, have made us more interested in . . . "the artifice, in and of itself." Consequently, what we want from stars is not their autographs. What we really want is what my friend Libby wanted during that lunch at Barney's—the names of their plastic surgeons.

Four

FINDING DR. RIGHT

*"Patients think beautiful hands are important. It's not the hands, it's the way
the surgeon thinks and sees. Hands are just the instrument of the brain."*
—YVES-GERARD ILLOUZ, THE FRENCH SURGEON
WHO POPULARIZED LIPOSUCTION

There are more than 150 board-certified plastic surgeons in New York
City alone and at least a dozen with world-class reputations. How do you
choose among titans? That was the problem I was confronted with when
I went shopping for my first face-lift—and what you will face when
choosing a surgeon. I want to take you through that experience because
there is much to be learned from it still—even without knowing the
names of the doctors.

Comparing recommendations from my dermatologist with those of
the always opinionated beauty underground, I make appointments with
four "Park Avenue" surgeons. Let's call the doctors W, X, Y, and Z.

My first consultation is with Dr. W, a man rumored to have operated
on a former First Lady. Like many novices shopping for a face-lift, I felt a
bit intimidated and wondered if a prominent doctor would give me an
appointment without a "reference." So I asked an acquaintance to call
ahead and smooth the way. I have since learned that it's not necessary to
have connections to get an appointment—although, I may have been seen
sooner because my friend made the call.

I ask J, my husband, to keep me company. "I'm just doing research," I
insist. He's not fooled for a minute.

Dr. W's softly lit waiting room is done in a contemporary style.
Camel-colored sectionals line facing walls, and there is no place for coats.

I get a form: Name, Address, Occupation ("Journalist," I write, as I will at all my appointments. There is no point in being dishonest). Insurance (irrelevant, since the cosmetic aspects of aging are not covered by any medical plan). Do you smoke? ("Quit smoking thirty years ago.") Etc. The consultation fee is 150 dollars, to be paid in advance.

After twenty minutes, we are led (lugging our coats) to a modern treatment room. J. uneasily scans the medical paraphernalia on the counter. Finally, the doctor, dynamic and professorial, enters and shakes hands. I'd imagined he'd ask me about my life and my work, why I wanted this. I'd imagined I'd tell him it wasn't to save my marriage. I am absolutely certain my husband wouldn't leave me because of a sagging chin (of course, he doesn't mind if I look good). I'd imagined I would say I hate the stranger in the mirror. And then I'd imagined, the doctor would tell me I was an attractive woman who couldn't benefit from his talents.

In my dreams! There is no such conversational foreplay. If the doctor-patient interview is a "mutual selection process," Dr. W must be reading the bumps on my skull or asking his questions telepathically.

Dr. W directs me to stand in front of a small mirror over a washbasin: "Let's see what you need." He grabs the flesh of my upper eyelid and pronounces it "crepey. We can cut that out. The lower lid is not bad, but we can take a little out."

Next, the neck.

"Lord, you haven't seen your jawline in years," he says. "We can take all that fat out, do a little liposuction under your chin. Tighten the neck muscles, pull up the cheeks. You'll look great. We could raise the forehead, but you'd have a surprised look. Not necessary. You need the classic face-lift. Eyes, face, neck."

He groans when I pull out a picture, expecting the kind of movie-star photo many prospective patients foist on doctors in this specialty. But it's a heavily retouched head shot of myself taken four years ago. "You won't look that good," he warns. I like his honesty, but it doesn't give me much incentive to take the next step.

"Come into my office and we can discuss it comfortably," he says. Silhouetted in front of a wall of textbooks, he gives what seems to be an oft-repeated rundown: "We do it in the hospital under general anesthesia. I have the best anesthesiologist in New York. No complications in nine thousand procedures. You wake up. Your head is in a foam helmet. No constriction. No pain. You stay twenty-four to forty-eight hours. The only problem: those little lines on your upper lip."

Dr. W offered two tried-and-true alternatives for the lip. "We could paint the area with acid," he says, "but you get some skin bleaching you may not like. I prefer to use dermabrasion—that's the only thing that hurts. My wife had it. She said she'd never talk to me again if I told patients it was no worse than a bad sunburn. It burns for a day or two. You can take a little Tylenol."

I tell him I'm not sure I want to go through dermabrasion. Meanwhile I'm trying to figure out which beauty in the silver-framed photo facing us is his wife and which is his daughter.

"Think about it, he says, "the lift will last twelve to fifteen years." This, as it turns out in my case, was overly optimistic. "The eyes will last about eight years." This wasn't optimistic enough. "The neck will never look this bad again. Once you remove the fat cells, they won't come back. Complications are very rare. Blood clots can come from spikes in blood pressure. We don't allow your pressure to get that high."

He can't say exactly how long the numbness in my face will last—a month, six months, a year? "Just know this: The feeling always comes back."

When he describes where the incisions will be, he's not interested in seeing my ropey appendectomy scar. "The face heals better than any part of the body," he scoffs. This statement stuns me. It means that everything my mother told me about my tendency to scar badly was wrong. I could have a successful face-lift. Suddenly I see, this journalistic inquiry can be a real, personal possibility. Perhaps not with this person, though. I find his bedside manner to be more than a little lacking.

"If you decide to go ahead with it," he says, "you'll come back the week beforehand so I don't have to recall what you look like after eight months." I can see his point, but it makes me feel forgettable. But then comes the kicker: "Oh, yes," he says. "You'll have to stop smoking." Has he been paying any attention to me at all?

"I stopped smoking thirty years ago," I remind him. "I wrote it on the card."

He looks again. "Excellent," he chirps. "Smoking is very bad. Nice to meet you," he says, dismissing us into the hands of a chatty nurse for further questions and prices. Often, it's the nurses who decide whether the patient is an impossible-to-please perfectionist, a plasti-surgiholic or overly acquiescent. One West Coast surgeon asks his patients to fill out a psychological questionnaire, designed to ferret out problem types. If patients refuse, he won't treat them.

Dr. W's grand total for face, neck, eyes, and lip peel: $18,500 (plus hospital, private nurses, and anesthesia). At those prices, I told my husband later, Dr. W should think about installing a coat closet.

The Ritual Search

I like to think I'm the sort of person who would choose a surgeon rationally, but when all things are equal, observed Harvard plastic surgery professor Robert M. Goldwyn, the choice of doctor is made "more on the basis of trust than of knowledge." That's why impression management—marble floors, slick brochures, receptionists that look like Vanna White—play a subliminal role in the selection process. If you don't like the painting on the wall (or the nonexistent coat closet), you may question the surgeon's aesthetic judgment. And if the doctor's hair is dyed a bizarre color or the chandeliers are over the top, he or she may be Dr. Wrong—for you. Taste is the great match-maker, said French sociologist Pierre Bourdieu. It brings people together, doctors and patients as well as husbands and wives.

No one can choose a doctor for you. It's important to do your own interviewing and to feel comfortable with your choice.

You may obsess about a face-lift, talk about it in the abstract to friends, and clip "before-and-after" articles from magazines, but it's all window-shopping until you make an appointment for a consultation. Meeting face-to-face with a surgeon, you can admit your dissatisfactions and your fears, find out if your expectations are realistic and get a real sense of the cost and how you relate to the person. Having a consultation doesn't mean you have to sign up for surgery, any more than *trying on a* dress means you have to buy it. But if you're prone to making impulse purchases, don't get near the office of someone who doesn't have confirmed *bona fides*.

Samantha, a West Coast magazine editor, rued the day she responded to an article in a tabloid about Gore-Tex lip enhancement. "On a lark," she consulted the doctor featured in the story. She never intended to actually *have* the surgery. But the doctor said he had a cancellation the next day and could work her in. He promised that anything she didn't like about the surgery could be easily fixed. As it turned out, she didn't like *anything* about it: she couldn't speak well; her lips looked grotesque; and she developed an infection. And, unfortunately, it couldn't be fixed. The doctor admitted he had never removed Gore-Tex before. Samantha paid dearly for his inexperience. Her upper lip is thinner than before, and uneven, and she suffered permanent sensory loss.

I imagine that the worst feeling in the world is being wheeled into an operating room and wondering, "Maybe I should have done more research on this." After all, even vacuum cleaner salesmen give you a few days to change your mind.

Diploma Confusion

Today anyone with an M.D. degree—even general practitioners, gynecologists, and urologists—can call themselves cosmetic surgeons and perform any operation they want to in a private office. And they want to more and more. That's where the money is since the country's move to managed care has put a lid on fees for reimbursable procedures. Cosmetic surgery is virtually the only field in which surgery is almost entirely elective and patients pay for the services, out of pocket, in advance. This is just one more factor that makes finding a doctor daunting.

There's a common fantasy about the perfect plastic surgeon, the one who's in demand, but available on short notice; compassionate, attentive, a wizard with scars, but so meticulous he or she does only one face-lift a day—because art can't be rushed; and reasonably priced, but not to the point of being the lowest bidder. "Dawn," a high-powered financial consultant, proudly admitted she had gone hunting for someone to remake her not long ago. And where had this search begun? With her hairdresser, of course.

Why is it that when we need an appendectomy, we'll take the advice of our family doctor, but when we need a face-lift we'll ask a beautician? "Any sensible woman knows that her hairdresser knows more about face-lifts than her GP," as Norma Lee Browning put it in her 1981 book *Face-lifts: Everything You Always Wanted to Know*, "and anyone who tries to tell you differently is daffy."

Then call me daffy.

Theoretically, hairdressers know who *had* it done, who *did* it to whom, and who *redid* it later. But I've heard beauticians trash some surgeons with excellent reputations and praise some questionable ones. Sometimes, it's a difference of taste, and sometimes, perhaps, recommendations are influenced by financial considerations. Three months after a beautician insisted Dr. So-and-so was the greatest, the same beautician proudly showed me her new nose done—actually, overdone—by that very same doctor. She didn't mention whether she'd gotten a break on the price and I didn't ask. But suffice to say, hairdressers aren't infallible.

One would think that the wives of doctors would have an easier job finding a good plastic surgeon than the rest of us, but several doctors' wives I know have refused their husbands' advice on the subject of cosmetic surgeons.

"Laurel," forty-nine, is married to a cancer specialist on the staff of a major teaching institution. Laurel hated her double chin. "I ski and I wear turtlenecks," she said. "My neck and jowls are hitting my turtleneck and it makes me crazy. I was never obsessed with my looks. I don't want to change them. I just want fine tuning."

Laurel knows many women who have had face-lifts. She rates some of the work "too tight" and some "not tight enough." She laughed at the suggestion that she ask her suburban family physician for a referral. "He'd just send you to his friends. I want the best." Laurel's husband, meanwhile, couldn't imagine why anyone, especially his wife, would want surgery she didn't need, but he wanted to be supportive so he selected a surgeon he knew by reputation and accompanied Laurel to the consultation. They were kept waiting for an hour and a half, and then the surgeon wouldn't show before and after pictures—which annoyed Laurel.

This is a complex issue. Many reputable doctors refuse to show before and after pictures. Not only can they be easily faked, says Michael Kane, M.D., a young New York plastic surgeon who doesn't use them, they are misleading. "Say, I've done a hundred rhinoplasties and I have to select one or two before-and-after pictures to show," says Kane. "I'm not going to pick the *average* good rhinoplasty. It's just human nature, I'm going to pick the *single best*, or the *two best* results. That's not really right." Instead of pictures, some doctors will introduce you to other patients who have had a similar operation.

After the first consultation, Laurel's husband told her she was on her own. It took a year of searching, but Laurel eventually settled on a young but well-trained surgeon discovered by a friend and she is pleased with the results. Now she has entered the king-making stage—justifying her choice by steering friends to her doctor. Satisfied patients often become evangelists for their favorites.

"Janine," an independent type in Dallas, however, is skeptical of advice from bosom buddies. "Girlfriends," says Janine, a restaurant manager, "tend to exaggerate, whether it's 'Use this shampoo,' or 'Go to this doctor.' " Janine found her doctor through his advertisement on the Internet. She was impressed with his curriculum vitae.

Celebrities are walking before-and-afters. If they don't know who's best, it's assumed, who does? People want to know: Who did that living legend and who did the star who looks like a perpetual teenager? Many wanted the name of Phyllis Diller's surgeon, as if that would be a guarantee of good results. (In fact, Diller, who, as I pointed out in the last chapter, did as much as anyone to fuel the plastic surgery explosion in the 1970s, has been operated on by several surgeons.)

Another kind of word-of-mouth—and a highly influential one—that can boost a doctor's reputation, is a mention in a magazine. Doctors, like any other professional who depends on client self-referrals, will sometimes pay thousands of dollars a month to press agents who can get their names in magazines. And women, the prime market for plastic surgery, are particularly vulnerable to what they read in magazines when contemplating changes in appearance. A Yankelovich study found that when women are thinking of making an image change they head for the newsstand in droves; 41 percent of women eighteen to forty-nine and 51 percent of the over-forty group leaf through magazines for ideas.

Nancy, a marketing executive pushing fifty, for example, has a page reserved in her Filofax for plastic surgeons' names. She doesn't need their services yet but is anticipating the day when she wakes up and her face has suddenly fallen. Whenever she reads or hears something favorable about someone new, she adds the name to her list for future reference.

Media validation has become such an important source of referrals that some physicians—in their handouts to patients—will list magazines and TV shows where they have been mentioned. One surgeon I've heard about keeps scrapbooks of his clippings in his waiting room to impress both patients and prospects.

But fashion magazines are not peer-reviewed journals. The doctor mentioned may be excellent, but he may also be the one with the most aggressive press agent.

"When I see on a patient's chart, 'referred by a magazine article,' I tell the patient, 'That's a terrible way to choose a doctor,' " says New York plastic surgeon Daniel C. Baker. "Patients should be referred by a personal physician. What's most important is [a surgeon's] reputation with other physicians." Baker notes, however, that personal references are valuable. "If three friends went to him and they all look good, that's important too."

"Hally," a pacing horse for her Tampa friends, used a combination of recommendations—from her hairdresser, from her dermatologist, and from a retired plastic surgeon friend—before choosing a doctor. Very few of Hally's friends have had face-lifts, and those who have won't talk about it. "Once I announced I was going to start the interview process and I'd likely have the surgery done in six months to a year after I completed my study, everyone wanted to know how you go about finding a doctor," says Hally, who wanted a full face-lift, an eye-lift, and her droopy upper lid repaired. As part of the selection process, she asked each doctor what else he would suggest. All suggested chin augmentation as well, something

Hally hadn't even considered as a possibility. (A chin implant for a weak chin is one of the few procedures plastic surgeons feel it is ethical to suggest if the patient doesn't ask about it.) Three of the four surgeons suggested bringing in an oculo-plastic specialist to repair her eyelid. The doctor she chose—the one recommended by her plastic surgeon friend—won on three counts. First, he described how subtle changes in the height of one side of her brow could balance her face better. Second, he was the only one who said he could hide the scar so she could wear her hair pulled back. And third, Hally liked his personality best. "I wanted someone I could get along with."

Hally was one of the very few people who, for no apparent reason, develop a hematoma ten days after surgery. The doctor and his staff were extremely attentive, and Hally chalked it up to fate. Now that the problem has cleared up, Hally has enthusiastically referred friends to him.

Doctors know that the majority of patients they see are making the rounds. I've heard of one patient that had sixteen consultations before settling on a surgeon. At one hundred to four hundred dollars per consult, it can add up, but think of it this way: How many cars would you test-drive before buying a new one? How many architects would you interview before building a house?

Reading the Signs

My second consultation is with the up-and-coming Dr. X. I've heard he is developing a loyal following among savvy young professionals. My husband is again by my side. ("I don't want you to think I'm encouraging this, but I want to give you moral support," he says.) The spacious waiting room is designed with a Capital D. There is a large coat closet with matching hangers, sofas covered in trendy tapestry, flattering lighting, and, on one wall, one of those landscape paintings that sell for $8,000 in SoHo galleries. On an end table, an engraved brass sign admonishes: *No Eating or Drinking in the Waiting Room.* In blatant disregard someone has left an open Diet Coke can with a lipstick-tipped straw. Is it significant to my future care that this blemish is being ignored?

During our hour-long wait, some of the staff, sitting behind a high counter, ignore us while bantering loudly among themselves. "I'd never trust a doctor who hired these people," grumps my husband. He's not off the mark. Getting a good feeling from the doctor's staff is important. If the doctor has a busy practice, and your surgery goes well, you will have more contact with the staff than with the doctor. Finally, after another twenty-minute wait in an examining room, the doctor arrives.

I like him and his approach. Not until he has gone over my medical history in detail does he look at my face. "Tell me," he says, "what don't you like when you look in the mirror?"

"My profile," I say, "my chin."

"That's the most common complaint. That can be taken care of," he says, putting his hands on my face for the first time. "A little lipo under the chin."

"I also don't like the sagging jowls."

"A classic face-lift can take care of that," he says, pulling up my cheeks. "The eyes aren't bad, just need a tiny tuck above and a little lipo below. How do you feel about the lip?" he asks. "We can take care of that with a little dermabrasion or a peel. That's the only thing you won't like. The face-lift feels a little tight at first, but you shouldn't have much pain. The lip on the other hand . . ."

I stop him. "I don't want the lip," I tell him. "I've seen women whose skin looks a different color on the lip."

"Good decision," he says. "I try to talk people out of it, hang the black crepe, but some people can't stand any wrinkles. You can't go wrong by doing less." Later, I regretted not exploring lip options with him. Would I have been more disposed to him if he had tried to educate me? But reputable doctors do not push you into procedures you don't want.

I tell him I fear the pulled-up look. Most of the time, he says, that's the result of multiple operations. When I show him my trusty retouched picture of myself, he says, "That's how you'll look. I can give you a decade." My pulse starts racing. Even my husband seems momentarily impressed. We talk about the downside. Far down. Death could occur (it's surgery, after all) but it's extremely rare under these circumstances. There's also a remote chance of nerve damage. Without looking, I know my husband has turned pale. Me, too.

After a generous forty-five minutes, Dr. X turns us over to his office manager who shows us before and after pictures that don't influence me one way or another. Dr. X's fee is a lot less than Dr. W's—$12,500 for the face, neck and eyes. I'm given printed material and advised to schedule surgery one month in advance. Consultation fee: $100. Dr. X is a possibility—although over the next few weeks, I become more curious about treatments for the lip and begin to explore options by talking to friends who have undergone them.

The Credential Dilemma

All of the doctors I consulted were board-certified plastic surgeons, but board certification is a quagmire. The question I ask when I look at all those claims of board certification in Yellow Pages ads is: Board certified in what specialty? And by whom? I don't want a board-certified urologist doing my face-lift. Trying to explain medical boards is like Abbott & Costello doing Who's On First? So pay attention.

Under the rules of the American Medical Association (AMA), each medical specialty has a certifying board. This board sets the standards of training (how many years of school, residency, etc.) and administers the annual written and oral exams that earn a specialist "board certification" in his or her specialty.

There is only one organization in this country recognized by the AMA for accrediting medical specialists: *The American Board of Medical Specialties (ABMS)*, located in Evanston, Illinois. The ABMS accredits physicians in twenty-four specialties from the American Board of Allergy & Immunology to the American Board of Urology. (See the list of the twenty-four ABMS boards on page 219.)

Yet, at last count there were 130 "self-designated" (some people call them "bogus") boards, each with official sounding names. One extra word in a board name could represent the difference between a doctor having seven years of specialized training or having taken no more than a weekend course.

There is no ABMS board with the word "cosmetic" in its title. Only two ABMS boards, the "American Board of Plastic Surgery" and the

"American Board of Otolaryngology"—ear, nose, and throat treatment or E.N.T. for short—certify doctors who perform surgical face-lifts. But nine of the 130 "self-designated" boards have the words "plastic," "facial," or "cosmetic" in their titles. All use the prefix "American Board of" before such designations as Cosmetic Plastic Surgery; Cosmetic Surgery; Facial Cosmetic Surgery; Facial Plastic Surgery; Head Facial & Neck Pain & TMJ Orthopedics; Int'l Cosmetic & Plastic Facial Reconstructive Standards; Laser Surgery; Otorhinolaryngology; Maxillofacial Surgeons; Plastic Aesthetic Surgeons; Skin Specialists.

Consumers need sharp eyes to separate the genuine sheepskins from the naugahyde ones. The Medical Board of California voted in July 1997 that doctors in the state can no longer advertise that they are "board-certified cosmetic surgeons" since the training curriculums of the American Board of Cosmetic Surgery (ABCS) do not match those of an ABMS board. The ruling is being contested by the ABCS.

Surgeons accredited by the American Board of Plastic Surgery are accredited to work on every part of the body and do everything from tumor removal to breast reconstruction to face-lifting. Currently, there are 5,335 board-certified plastic surgeons in the U.S. (1,250 of whom concentrate on aesthetic surgery).

The advent of antibiotics and the decline in ear and nose infections have led otolaryngologists (E.N.T. specialists) to branch out. Besides rhinoplasties (nose jobs) which they have always done, many E.N.T. specialists now perform face-lifts. They are accredited by the American Board of Otolaryngology. (While they often call themselves facial-plastic surgeons, there is no ABMS board of facial plastic surgery.)

Ophthalmologists can also do cosmetic procedures, notably eye-lifts. They are certified by the American Board of Ophthalmology. Some eye doctors call themselves "oculo-plastic surgeons" although there is no ABMS board of oculo-plastic surgery. But a surgeon may be "double-boarded"—that is have boards in two specialties: say, ophthalmology and plastic surgery.

Dermatologists are certified by the American Board of Dermatology (another bonafide ABMS board). Dermatology is not considered a surgical specialty in medical schools, and, unless they take extra training in surgery, dermatologists do not usually have operating privileges at hospi-

tals. However, many dermatologists now call themselves "surgical dermatologists" (although there is no ABMS board of surgical dermatology). In
addition to skin peels and excision of tumors and lesions, some dermatologists now do liposuction and blepharoplasties (eye-lifts)—and by the
year 2000, they may be doing face-lifting too, an issue which will only
get more controversial.

Warns one plastic surgeon, "There is nothing to stop anyone from
incorporating as, say, the Board of Face-Lift Surgery. You could sell cer-
tificates for $1,000 and the people who bought them could say they were
board-certified by this entity. They're not lying. But the credential is
meaningless."

Boards are different from societies. *Societies* and *associations* are political and educational organizations, *not* certifying bodies. (Usually, though,
a physician can't join a society without being a member of the related
board.) Societies and associations hold scientific meetings and give
courses. It's important for surgeons who practice cosmetic surgery to
attend scientific meetings regularly. Plastic surgery is a dynamic field
with constant innovation. You want a doctor who keeps up with
advances. As Frank McDowell, an early plastic surgeon wrote, "You have
to learn what others have done because you won't live long enough to
make all the mistakes yourself."

Most of the 5,335 board-certified plastic surgeons belong to the
American Society of Plastic and Reconstructive Surgeons (ASPRS).
ASPRS members who concentrate on aesthetic surgery may also belong
to the American Society for Aesthetic Plastic Surgery (ASAPS), which
has 1,250 members. Both these societies have toll-free numbers and web-
sites to assist consumers in finding qualified surgeons. (See page 218 for
addresses and telephone numbers.)

Many of the board-certified otolaryngologists who do face-lifting
and other cosmetic procedures belong to the American Association of
Facial Plastic and Reconstructive Surgeons (AAFPRS). I reiterate, AAF-
PRS is not a board, but board certification in otolaryngology or plastic
surgery is required for membership.

Another test of legitimacy is whether the doctor has operating privileges *for the procedure* you're contemplating—say, endoscopic brow-
lifting—at an accredited hospital. Even the chief of plastic surgery has to

take the necessary courses and earn the certificate in endoscopy before being allowed to use an endoscope in the hospital. But doctors who operate in their own offices can use any equipment they please, even without the necessary courses.

Of course, board certification, society memberships, and hospital privileges are just starting points. All they guarantee is that the doctor has the necessary basic training: a medical degree, three years of approved general surgical training, an accredited two- or three-year residency in the specialty, at least two years in practice, and has passed oral and written exams, and has a place to conduct business. Board certification does not guarantee a perfect result.

CeCe, the thirty-one-year-old actress I met in Arizona, found her doctor in a medical library. "I was such a regular [at a local medical library]," says CeCe, "I would call ahead and the clerk would have the directories of medical specialists waiting for me when I arrived." CeCe interviewed ten surgeons before she settled on one. "I was as educated as any layperson could be prior to going into surgery." But still, while she was very happy with her brow lift, she was unhappy with her liposuction and had it redone.

"The greatest surgeons in the world have complications and patients who require touch-ups. Anyone who claims not to have problems is not telling the truth," says one prominent surgeon. But a competent surgeon knows how to treat them, and will be there for the patient should problems occur.

Many specialists in the field like to stress their artistic credentials in their ads or their press releases. It is debatable whether the quality of a doctor's artwork correlates to surgical talent. As one plastic surgeon told me facetiously, "There are more great artists in plastic surgery than there were in Italy in the fifteenth century." A West Coast press agent, for example, straining credibility, promotes one client, a cosmetic surgeon who is a board-certified otolaryngologist, as the "Michelangelo of his profession." The accompanying photo of the doctor shows him wearing a necktie painted with the torso of a bimbo. Dubious.

The confusion about doctors has even spawned a new field—the cosmetic-surgery matchmaker. Judith Cohen, a psychologist with experience in direct marketing is the proprietor of "1-800-Beautify," a plastic surgery information hotline serving California and the Phoenix area. Cohen and her ten-person staff field up to hundreds of calls a week from consumers, gratis. Surgeons she has investigated and invited to be members of her club pay monthly dues to swim in what are in many ways very choppy waters.

According to laws in some states, it is a misdemeanor for doctors to give or get money for referring a patient. One doctor can send a patient to another doctor but he's not allowed to take any money for it. (Even a case of wine at Christmas is frowned on, although they are still being sent and received.) A matchmaker can't get money from a doctor for a referral either—although if she were on the doctor's staff she could receive a bonus for talking a patient into surgery. "That's the equivalent of Nordstroms paying a salesperson a commission," says plastic surgeon Ronald E. Iverson, former president of the ASPRS. "The patient is not being misled. Patients know they're dealing with an employee. At least it's up front."

Doctors are, however, permitted to advertise and avail themselves of public relations and referral services, as long as it's made clear to the public whom the matchmaker represents. "For ten years, we worried about truth in advertising," says Iverson. Now, with the rise of referral services, he says, there's "a new level of ethical dilemma."

Choosing a doctor has never been an easy decision, but with all "the friendly advice" out there from press agents, hairdressers, and matchmakers (not to mention friends who want to justify their own choices), prospective patients now have to also figure out if the so-called patient advocates aren't really *doctor* advocates. It would be nice if there were one perfect way to find a doctor. The truth is that there are a wealth of sources for recommendations, but none of them can be relied upon exclusively. Credentials matter. But so does reputation, taste, experience in the procedure in question, and results that can be verified, preferably by satisfied patients.

Reading—or Misreading—the Signs

I go alone for my consultation with Dr. Y (my husband is out of town). His office is country-club traditional—wing chairs and Chippendalia. I can't explain why, but I feel slightly intimidated. Is it because the two secretaries stationed behind a high mahogany counter seem to be giving me the once-over? Or is it that the women in the waiting room look like they walked over from lunch at Harry Cipriani. That's no crime. I eat there too, now and then.

Dr. Y's form is the first that asks Husband's Occupation; is this significant? I suppose it's mostly the husbands who pay the bills for this surgery. After a short wait, I am shown into an old-fashioned but spotless treatment room. On one wall hangs a framed news story about Dr. Y. After twenty minutes, the gray-haired doctor arrives in a tidy white coat. He is polite and professional—not slick, but not-country doctor warm either. I am predisposed to like him: He has a fine reputation and many devotees. He takes a comprehensive medical history but doesn't seem interested in me personally. This puts me off. Much later I realize he's more shy than standoffish.

When I produce my wannabe photo, he says, no problem, "I can take ten years off your face." Handing me a brass mirror, he uses a slim metal implement to show me what he would take out of my upper eyelid. Then the lower eyelid. Then he takes my cheek and raises it up gently while tucking my chin under—to show the effect I'd get. "You'll still have the smile lines, but not so deep. You won't be pulled tight. You won't lose your expression. And you should have a peel or dermabrasion on your upper lip." I hesitate, saying I have seen women with bleached-looking upper lips. "You'll regret not doing it," he says sternly, without allaying my fears or explaining further. "You might as well do it all at once."

He may be right, but he doesn't convince me. He assures me I'll have no problem healing and passes me on to the fee lady. Eyes: $6,000. Face and neck: "$10,000. Dermabrasion: $1,000. Done all together: $15,000, plus hospital charges. (If I couldn't afford such fees, I would still have the consultation and ask for the recommendation of a protégé who might charge less.)

As I warm to the idea of a lift, I try the idea out on others in my extended family. "I wish I had done it when I was younger," my mother says. "But you don't need it," she adds diplomatically. And she raises the issue again about scarring.

Daughters, I've since found, have a hard time accepting a mother's lift. They want mom-the-nurturer, not mom-the-competitor. And my stepdaughters react true to form. They have another reason to be dismayed. Their mother died of a brain tumor. "Why do something painful and risky?" rails the youngest. "Shut up and grow old gracefully."

My son doesn't try to talk me out of it—perhaps because, as a photographer, he has seen the truth of my concerns in his lens, and because, as the son of a surgeon, he respects the specialty.

My son-in-law, an orthopedic resident at this time, is offended that I didn't ask for his recommendations on physicians. "Famous doctors aren't always good," he warns. Where have I heard that before?

When women trust the advice of their friends more than that of a physician, it reinforces the stereotype that women are impulsive and whimsical in their decisions. In matters of plastic surgery, however, there are extenuating circumstances.

I've assembled scrapbooks of articles about cosmetic surgery, dating back to the early 1900s. Leafing through them, it's easy to trace society's changing attitudes toward practitioners. For decades, family doctors judged women who wanted cosmetic surgery to be vain and neurotic, and the doctors who would do such work "charlatans," leaving the field to poorly trained practitioners who often promised more than they could deliver. The woman dissatisfied with her appearance was as easy a mark for self-promoters as her grandmother was for the huckster selling Lydia Pinkham's Vegetable Compound.

In 1925, a "self-confessed [beauty surgery] faker" admitted—anonymously—in *Liberty* magazine how, with limited medical training, but "with a graciousness that inspired confidence," he "fleeced and sometimes disfigured hundreds of women who came to him in the eternal feminine quest of loveliness."

The scoundrel's three-part confession recounted how plastic surgery emerged as a heroic specialty at the end of World War I and how the rogue, himself, took a course and opened an office, conning patients with the claim that he was trained in Europe. All he had to do, he said, was "tell them that Doctor So-and-so of Paris or Berlin has done the faces of the European nobility and that you learned your profession under him. Then watch them run to your office!"

He described his patients as "the veiled society woman, the bold-faced actress, and the shrinking young girl" and was astonished that "well-educated and thoroughly sophisticated [people never] thought of consulting some reputable surgeon." The money was good, he said, because "cosmetic surgery . . . has caused a certain hysteria among the homely and the aged and even the beautiful."

The knave admitted to tricks of the trade that are still in use today: falsifying before-and-after pictures; displaying photos of stage and screen stars and pretending they were patients; and leaking the news that "I operated on the prominent Mrs. Dwiddle-Dinks." He said the public's gullibility astonished him. "If you're thinking of going to a beauty surgeon," he advised, "consult your own doctor first. Otherwise you're liable to fall into the hands of a quack who'll wreck, at one stroke, both your good looks and your pocketbook."

The author of this tell-all may well have been the original Doctor Wrong, Henry Junius Schireson, king of the scoundrel-surgeons, and vain enough to want to boast of his deceits. With only a few medical courses to his credit and forged credentials, he established himself as a cosmetic surgeon in Chicago at the end of the World War I. In his thirty-year career, he was repeatedly arrested, convicted, sentenced, and jailed. After being banned from working in Chicago, Detroit, Pittsburgh, and New York, he moved to Philadelphia, where he built a booming practice by attending society functions and ingratiating himself to wealthy women with gifts of pedigreed puppies. Schireson got the most mileage out of two patients, Fanny Brice, whose nose job is believed to have been one of the doctor's publicity stunts, and the English actress Lady Diana Manners. He also boasted that he had worked on world champion prize-fighter Jack Dempsey's battered nose—although this was a popular claim among cosmetic surgeons of the day.

Unscrupulous doctors benefited from the American Medical Association's policy, which considered it unethical for a reputable doctor to have his name in print. Women were in a bind. The only names widely known were those who advertised or had press agents. So women gravitated to these unprincipled doctors.

As acceptance of cosmetic procedures increased, so did the admonitions. Lois Mattox Miller's 1939 article in *Independent Woman* (condensed a month later in *Readers' Digest*) warned that "plastic surgery is safe only in direct ratio to the skill of the surgeon. Beware charlatans and quacks who offer to transform the ugly duckling into a swan. . . . Ill-advised attempts at 'face-lifting' by quack surgeons have left untold numbers of women gruesomely scarred about the face and neck, their prized 'good looks' . . . ravaged." To illustrate this, she cited the most famous medical fiasco of the period—the Peaches Browning case.

Browning, a darling of the tabloids, was adopted as a child by industrialist A. B. Browning, who married her when she was fourteen. As she grew up, she developed heavy legs and wanted them thinned. She consulted (whom else?) Dr. Henry Schireson. He may or may not have been aware that fat removal in the legs had been tried in France in February 1926, with devestating results. The patient was a French model, Mme. Goeffre, who wanted to open a couture house. Skirts were getting shorter and she had thick legs. She consulted the respected Parisian orthopedist, Louis Charles Dujarier, who wasn't anxious to operate. He gave in when she threated to kill herself. During the surgery, a major blood vessel was injured, leading to gangrene and the amputation of one of the model's legs.

Peaches Browning lost *both* legs. Consequently, Schireson was arrested and spent three years in Leavenworth Penitentiary.

Beauty restoration had some good word of mouth, too. Plastic surgery was credited, perhaps undeservedly, with saving the face of the beautiful eighteen-year-old debutante, Barbara Cushing. In 1934, Babe, as she was known, the future Mrs. William S. Paley, was injured in a car crash. According to one biography, her face was "smashed almost beyond recognition and most of her teeth were knocked out. It took months of reconstructive surgery . . . but she emerged as beautiful as she had ever been, despite having to wear false teeth."

Though this success story may have boosted plastic surgery's profile, it may have also been an exaggeration. Thomas Rees, the Beautiful People's favorite New York plastic surgeon in the eighties, did a face-lift on Babe Paley when she was much older. "Perhaps she lost her teeth but she didn't have her face reconstructed," says Rees. "I knew her well. She had no scars."

Not long after Babe Cushing's accident in 1937, the American Board of Plastic Surgery was formed to certify plastic surgeons, and—

no surprise—soon, the press began emphasizing the importance of credentials. *Good Housekeeping* advised readers wanting nose surgery in 1940 to consult their family doctor for a referral and put themselves in the hands of a "fine plastic surgeon backed by a first-class hospital." Still many reputable surgeons felt only the "nasally desperate" deserved help.

Flash forward to the sixties. Women began taking charge of their bodies. They became Weight Watchers in 1961, and feminists in 1963, when Betty Friedan's *The Feminine Mystique* sent shivers through suburban Jell-O molds, and Cosmo girls in 1965. Although most of the attention was on equal pay for equal work, there was an unaddressed empowerment women desired that is rarely noted in histories of the period: They wanted face-lifts without guilt. In June 1960, *Harper's Bazaar* put its imprimatur on the face-lift, and inadvertently changed the course of medicine in the U.S.

Touching off a major legal battle among already warring medical specialty groups, Geri Trotta's article concluded: "Some ear, nose, and throat men (otolaryngologists) feel qualified to perform nasal plastics . . . and no law can stop them."

E.N.T. specialists were "outraged." Many of the early giants in plastic and reconstructive surgery had started as nose specialists and felt they owned the face. One nose surgeon in New Orleans was so incensed, he attempted to have plastic surgery "banished as a specialty." The infighting caught the attention of the Federal Trade Commission (FTC), which subsequently spent years trying, unsuccessfully, to do away with medical boards altogether and settled instead for making the AMA do away with its injunction against physician advertising. But it was nine years before a reputable doctor dared allow his name to be mentioned in a magazine. When that doctor came forward, the world of plastic surgery changed forever.

Vogue's Diana Vreeland was among those itching for more frankness on the subject. She wanted to mention doctors by name and she was determined to publish close-ups of a face-lift. When she showed her staff graphic under-the-skin pictures she had commissioned for publication in August 1969, "one left immediately to throw up," she recalled in her memoir, *Allure*. "Others were gagging and carrying on. . . . It was *un-*

believable!" she crowed. (The pictures never ran in *Vogue*, only in her book.)

Just before the decade ran out, in *Vogue*'s October 1, 1969, issue, Vreeland finally broke the taboo against mentioning a plastic surgeon by name. The breakthrough article, written by Simona Morini, was called, "Body Sculpturing: New Techniques in Cosmetic Surgery for Every Part of the Body . . . and a Working Day in the Life of an Internationally Famous Doctor."

The story started dramatically:

"8 A.M. Dr. Ivo Pitanguy is enjoying his weekly massage in a small, bare room at his private clinic in Rio de Janeiro. High above his head he holds a small volume of Bertold Brecht's poems from which he reads aloud."

"That's when the roof fell off the building!" recalled Vreeland. "I mean the medical men were calling from all over the country. 'This is totally unethical. It's never been done before.' And I said, 'Well, it's high time! People want to know where they can get this done! What's the big secret? Aren't you in business?' "

Vogue labeled Pitanguy, "one of the most remarkable young . . . plastic surgeons in the world." And, most remarkable of all, while he courted publicity, he was no Schireson. He had impeccable medical credentials. It would take years for the medical establishment to accept the fact that publicity and charlatanism didn't necessarily go hand in hand.

Pitanguy was the Pygmalion that women—and not just American women—had been waiting for. Even before *Vogue* singled out Doctor Ivo, a samba had been written about him, and Rio taxi drivers knew he was "the man who irons out all Rio ladies' wrinkles." To say he attracted patients is an understatement. In him, the affluent found an eloquent apologist for their body obsessions in an exotic locale, surrounded by a whole category of people to emulate—"the Beautiful People." Even today, on Park Avenue, in Bel Air, or on Avenue Foch, women seeking cosmetic surgery wonder, Maybe I should be going to that guy in Brazil. Pitanguy, close to seventy, is still working, although he does only a part of each operation.

The American medical establishment was horrified by Pitanguy's public emergence. "The consequences [of self-promotion] were severe," recalls Tom Rees, who started practice in 1957. What Pitanguy's critics refused to acknowledge was that Pitanguy was different from the untrained schemers who had been preying on women since the 1920s. Pitanguy, the son of a surgeon, was a Renaissance man. Not only was he a sportsman, a cultured man who collected art and spoke five or six languages, he was well-trained and a talented surgeon.

Pitanguy decided to specialize in plastic surgery while treating World War II casualties during his general surgery residency in Cincinnati. But training programs in the specialty were virtually nonexistent in the 1950s. Doctors had to construct their own course of study and obtain fellowships with the small number of experts around the world. Many practitioners were secretive. Some even charged observers admission. Pitanguy obtained visiting fellowships with the leading reconstructive surgeons of the day—Paul Tessier in France, Sir Harold Gillies and Sir Archibald McIndoe in England—where Pitanguy met Rees.

Once, while watching Gillies do a face-lift, Pitanguy recalls, Gillies said something inspirational: "If I didn't think this had value, I wouldn't do it."

The defining moment in Pitanguy's career came in 1961 when a madman torched a circus tent in a town near Rio, trapping 2,500 people. Nearly four hundred people, mostly children, died the first day. Hundreds more had second- and third-degree burns. Pitanguy, who was chief of plastic surgery at three different hospitals in Rio, mobilized their care. "For three days and three nights," wrote Pitanguy in his autobiography, "we operated, grafted, nursed, and prayed."

He had an epiphany when one of the survivors, a young man, looked at his scarred face in a mirror and said, " 'I'd rather be dead.' At that moment," wrote Pitanguy, "I realized it was not enough to repair. I dedicated my life to beauty."

Soon, he launched a U.S.-style surgical residency program, vowing to let anyone observe and to make cosmetic surgery respectable. He was one of the few in the specialty who saw no difference between reconstructive and cosmetic procedures. He understood how films, television, and social and geographic mobility fueled dissatisfaction with appearance, inspiring women to emulate stars like Marilyn Monroe.

"Man has always sought to be similar to his peers, to his tribe and his social group," wrote Pitanguy. "Difference implies being ostracized." But the media and information bombardment "interferes with the perception of reality and has deep emotional consequences, [creating] impossible dreams. The individual aspires no longer to be like his peers, but rather to this group or that, whose economic and cultural supremacy has imposed their own image on him." Well-being, he said, is "the capacity to be in harmony and peace with [one's] own image."

By the mid-seventies, "going to Rio" had become a euphemism for checking into Pitanguy's seventeen-bed clinic for a face-lift or the innovative tummy tuck, buttocks lift, and breast-lift procedures he developed before liposuction supplanted many of his techniques. If Hollywood made the face-lift a secret vice, Pitanguy made it as glamorous as a Riviera holiday. Clinica Pitanguy became a magnet for film stars, society, and Europe's formerly titled—the rich and fabulous, from (it's rumored) Josephine Baker to Queen Farah Diba, and Gina Lollobrigida.

Eleanor Lambert, the founder of the International Best Dressed List, had an eyelift at Pitanguy's clinic and recalls what it was like to be a patient in his luxuriously appointed all-white rooms. "It was a slice of high life I had never seen before," she recalls. "A mix of Brazilians and women from around the world. Rich, spoiled women and butterflies. (And behind one closed door, a young boy, badly burned in a car crash.) There was a dormitory feeling. There was no attempt to hide or be prudish about it. It was like having your hair tinted. A ritual you go through."

Pitanguy understood instinctively what psychologists working with plastic surgery patients realized later: that plastic surgery can relieve depression and restore defenses in women with unresolved grief reactions. "Ivo has great tenderness for women who want to fulfill themselves," says Lambert. "There was a generosity to his idea that every woman had a right to look her best."

If American doctors indulged in the kind of self-promotion Pitanguy did, "they would have lost their licenses, been thrown out of the club," says Rees. (Actually, Pitanguy *was* thrown out of the club—in 1980. The ASPRS revoked his corresponding membership after a lengthy profile of him appeared in the *New York Times Magazine*. The photo of "Doctor

Vanity," bare-chested in his swim trunks, surrounded by a bikini-clad trio, drinking champagne on a speeding cigarette boat was the last straw for some colleagues who deemed it a "bad image for plastic surgery." Pitanguy was eventually reinstated. And when the AMA's ban on publicity was dropped in 1979, says Rees, "the world caught up with Ivo."

His legacy may be his ability to articulate the psychological value of the face-lift. "Not everyone ages equally well," he said on a recent visit to the U.S. Anti-aging surgery is "a positive act—to make aging less destructive, to make the transition from youth to maturity a happy one. But face-lifts for aging have to be subtle," he said. "You can't have total rejuvenation and still keep the integrity of the face. You want to recognize yourself." The goal is "to give age a dignified expression, a frame the spirit can inhabit—so you feel you will survive. With some people, you operate to give a person back to himself—to restore balance and energy. But on the wrinkles of the soul, we cannot operate."

Reading Is Not Believing

With the advent of advertising and publicity in the eighties, consumers needed more than ever to differentiate the qualified from the unqualified doctor. *Mademoiselle* warned readers that "there's no correlation between the level of a cosmetic surgeon's skill and his ability to advertise." The drumroll for board-certified plastic surgeons continued—along with a new crop of scare stories. *Newsweek* in 1988 coined the term "scalpel slaves," patients so addicted to the knife, they went from doctor to doctor demanding surgery. The same year, *Glamour* called attention to the phenomenon of the surgical redo in "The Cosmetic Surgery Boom"—reporting that many doctors devoted 5 to 25 percent of their practice to fixing the mistakes of "cut-rate quacks." If that wasn't scary enough, the magazine cautioned against putting too much stock in diplomas—even the bonafide ones: Certification by the American Board of Plastic Surgery does not necessarily guarantee first-rate medical skills—or emotional sensitivity."

As predicted, advertising had given plastic surgery, more than any other specialty, " 'a quasi-carnival atmosphere' of hucksterism." The most sobering reality check came in 1985, when self-promoter Richard Dombroff (a surgeon who was not board-certified), owner of a chain of Personal-Best plastic surgery clinics performing 5,000 operations a year, was investigated by New York State for operating without surgical gloves or sterile instruments and employing unlicensed physicians to operate for him. Dombroff eventually was sentenced to three months in jail and nine months of community service and lost his medical license.

Is it any wonder prospective patients are distrustful? The AIDS epidemic has added another layer of fear to the patient-doctor relationship. In 1985 a totally unfounded rumor (believed to have been started by competitors) that Tom Rees was dying of AIDS "was being repeated at some of the best hairdressers" (remember them?) in New York. Rees's practice went overnight from full tilt to zero. Before he could resuscitate his reputation, arthritis in his hands forced him to retire.

The recession of the early nineties and the tremendous influx of physicians from other specialties into cosmetic surgery has made the current scene even more competitive. While consumer demand is up, so is desperate self-promotion. Every night on the news one doctor or another is demonstrating the latest technique for wrinkle removal. Doctors pay publicists mightily to get this sort of coverage because, invariably, the guy shown operating on TV can expect his phone to ring off the hook the next day.

Dr. Right

On the morning of my fourth face-lift research consultation—my appointment with Dr. Z—I beg my husband to come with me one last time. "Why should I go?" he says. "These guys never talk to me." Grumbling, he agrees.

Dr. Z's long narrow waiting room looks faintly like something out of *Architectural Digest*, with Roman shades on the windows, banquettes, and a hanging Japanese screen. The cookies on the reception counter are no temptation to the well-dressed and well-disciplined bodies waiting—several of them accompanied by husbands. The closet is stocked with the by-now-familiar brass hangers. The secretaries are as solicitous as flight attendants. One serves tea to a waiting patient.

Finally after an hour's wait, it's my turn, and we are ushered into Dr. Z's spacious plum-and-blue office. The diplomas are grouped cleverly in two giant frames. The grand cherrywood desk, with no backlog of paperwork waiting, declares a fastidious owner. Enter a nurse to pre-interview me (I suspect it's a holding operation because the doctor is running late) and to describe the facility next door, where stitches are removed and makeup instruction is provided for the black-and-blue period. Onward, now, to a designer examining room with tasteful drawer pulls. I have to remind myself that the decorator doesn't do the operation.

By now my husband is nearly apoplectic about the wait. At last the doctor enters with a nurse. He is beyond dapper in a well-tailored navy suit, a 100-dollar red silk tie, and spiffy white-collared blue shirt that a valet must have spent an hour pressing. Dr. Z is not tall but he has a large presence, made larger by self-confidence as full-blown as his Ted Koppel-esque hair.

"Well, I see by your chart you have a nice life," says the doctor with easy charm. Then to my astonishment he asks my husband about himself. That small gesture establishes instant rapport. "I see you're a journalist," he says, turning to me. He is the first doctor to ask me for whom I write. "Oh, I like that magazine." (It's not that I want VIP treatment. I just want to be seen as an individual—not just another jowled "before" face.)

"Why are you here?" he wants to know.

"I hate my neck," I tell him. "I want to look like this picture of myself."

"Okay," he says. "Let me tell you what I can do for you. Hold this mirror." He puts his hands on my face like a healer. "We can take the fat out of the eyes, raise the cheeks, get rid of the chin. But now, the forehead. We could get rid of those wrinkles with a forehead-lift."

"I'd like to do less, not more," I tell him.

"Then you can forget the forehead. What about the lip?" he asks. "Do you want the small lines smoothed out?"

"What do you have in mind?" I ask.

"We can do a light peel," says Dr. Z. "You don't need a heavy peel or dermabrasion. A light TCA [trichloroacetic acid] peel isn't painful. You might have to do it again in a few years, but you'll like the results."

I feel myself moving from Maybe to Yes. I get the sense that I wouldn't feel as if I were intruding if I had to call him on a weekend with an emergency question. If you had asked me before this consultation what I wanted in a plastic surgeon, I would have insisted it wasn't a hand-holder. I thought of myself as results-oriented—but maybe I want more of a personal connection than I realized.

"Women often say, 'I don't care about a doctor's personality. I'm not looking for a dinner companion,' " says Wendy Lewis, a New York plastic surgery consultant who advises prospective patients. "But invariably, they're the ones who will cross a doctor off their list for being 'too cold.' "

The suppressed emotions of the past months bubble up. "I'm terribly conflicted about this," I say, as tears well up. "I want to do it, but my husband isn't in favor of it. My stepchildren are against it. And I have two terrible fears. One is that I will die on the operating table, which would be so humiliating—to die of a face-lift. And the other fear is that I'll look like one of those ladies with their faces pulled tight. I have seen many younger women with marvelous natural results. Can I hope to look that good?"

"First," says Dr. Z, "I can't tell you if you should have surgery. That's your decision. But I will say this: Do you think I want you dying on me? I don't want it any more than you do. You'll be in twilight sleep and monitored all the time. You won't remember anything and you won't feel a thing."

As for the tight look: "This is what we're going to do," says Dr. Z. "I'm going to have one of my patients call you—she's older than you, and you can see her results. Don't make any decision until you see her."

On to the fee lady. Face and neck: $10,000; eyes: $6,000. For the package: $15,000, peel included. I make a tentative date for surgery on the spot. I can't believe I am doing this.

My husband and I barely speak till we get home.

"So what did you think of him?" I ask.

"He's obviously a dandy and a super salesman. How do you know he's good?"

My son-in-law checks out Dr. Z's reputation with medical colleagues. A friend puts me in touch with some of his younger patients, both very satisfied. Finally I get a call from Dr. Z's older patient. She said she had two face-lifts by Dr. Z—one when she was sixty-six and another when she was seventy-four. "And I intend to do it again," she said. "I'm seventy-eight now and I look no older than sixty."

Frankly, I'm skeptical.

A few evenings later I have a chance to judge for myself when she stops by. "I could tell you needed reassurance," she says. I look at her in wonder. There are no bags under her eyes. No sagging jowls. Her chin and jaw are flawless. Yet she looks totally natural. She *could* pass for sixty.

"Impossible," agrees my stunned husband.

"I can see you're hooked," he says after she leaves.

Two days later, I confirm my surgery date with Dr. Z.

After my decision, you might think that all my friends would follow my lead, but it doesn't work that way. When a friend asked me for a recommendation, I shared the names of the four doctors I had consulted and suggested she meet them and decide for herself. She made exactly the same rounds as I did—and chose Dr. Y.

Five

LIFE AND DEATH DETAILS

"God is in the details."

—MIES VAN DER ROHE AND GUSTAVE FLAUBERT

Nearly five years later, when I call to schedule my "before" pictures for my nose surgery and brow lift, the receptionist at the photo studio says matter-of-factly, "Don't wear any makeup." I know that. After all, I've been down this road before. If I hadn't been so timid the first time, I might not be making the trip again.

A set of "before" pictures are as vital to the face-lift as X rays are to orthopedics, and for most people, making the appointment for those pictures is a turning point, one signifying that the flirtation is over. The countdown has begun. A commitment has been made, and not just because you often have to pay for the pictures. In the overall scheme of things, the cost (a hundred and seventy-nine dollars for a set of face-lift shots and seventy-nine dollars for a nose series—"afters" included) is negligible.

Beyond New York, "The Pictures" are often included in the surgeon's fee. "My patients are trying to contain costs," says plastic surgeon Lawrence N. Seifert, who has a photo studio in his L.A. office and takes all his own pictures. "Taking them myself helps me focus on what needs to be done."

But where I live, most face-lift operations begin with pictures taken by either David Price or at the Don Allen Studio—where I've been sent.

The studio is a short walk from Bloomingdale's, just off Park Avenue in an anonymous medical office building. As I wait to be buzzed in, I catch my reflection in the black Plexiglas paneling framing the studio's entrance. In the low light, I think, "Hey, maybe I don't look so bad." That thought vanished once I saw the finished pictures.

This studio has been a fixture of the Park Avenue plastic-surgery scene since 1950 when Allen (now retired) was a medical photographer at Manhattan Eye, Ear & Throat Hospital (MEETH). Some of the most famous faces in the world—actors, anchorpersons, politicians, and socialites—have smiled and grimaced for the camera here, although there is no photographic evidence that any of these sessions have occurred. No files are kept. All pictures—those of celebrities and average folks alike—go to the doctors. The only client photos on display are of cute kids (another specialty of the house). The only celebrity photo on hand is a vintage one of Jacqueline Kennedy (before she was married to Onassis) on the cover of Time. Jackie's face sits prominently atop a stack of magazines. Is this a sly tip of the hat to a woman rumored to be a former client?

Before and after pictures have a long and noble tradition in plastic surgery. One of the earliest uses of photography was for pre- and postoperative pictures of reconstructive procedures. During the Civil War, Gurdon Buck, a New York Hospital surgeon, used daguerreotypes to illustrate the hideous disfigurements wreaked on soldiers by cannon shells and the less than perfect repairs he was able to make. It took several wars and innumerable scientific and technical developments to arrive at today's high level of face-saving.

The no-makeup requirement is a necessary indignity. These photos aren't meant to flatter. They are blueprints of the existing facade, an essential tool for planning renovations that also serve as reference points during surgery when a patients' features may be distorted by such factors as anesthesia, inserted tubes, or the position of the head.

In Hollywood, it's not uncommon for aspiring actresses to refuse to take official "befores" for the same reason they use aliases. The theory: The less proof of surgical intervention, the better. Because of the importance of pictures to the planning and execution of procedures—and for legal reasons—many plastic surgeons refuse to work on anyone who resists being photographed.

Because of their brutal honesty, "before" pictures may be the most painful aspect of undergoing a face-lift. One can imagine the pictures as a plot hatched by doctors to convince us we need surgery. Make no mistake: If you're on the fence, the "befores" will push you over.

But, even if the light were softer, says Byron Dobell, a portrait painter, it would be typical to hate the pictures. It's a function of age and gender. After the age of fifty, women hate realistic depictions of themselves, he says. "They see themselves as ten years younger. If you paint a man at fifty, he doesn't complain, 'You made me look too old.' But if you paint a woman accurately, she says, 'I look too old.' " No wonder I succumbed to the magic words: "I can give you ten years."

I try to remind myself that my "before" pictures aren't destined to hang over the living-room sofa—just over the operating table—and, in time, perhaps, they'll end up in some musty medical library, waiting to be unearthed by twenty-second-century anthropologists who will marvel at the bizarre body practices of twentieth-century women.

At Don Allen's, the process of getting these pictures taken has all the charm of being detained in an interrogation chamber in a banana republic. My hair is bobby-pinned back. I'm told to remove my turtleneck sweater, which will hide my neck. I'm given a little terrycloth coverup for my chest. And I'm seated in a swivel chair in the center of the room, in front of a gray paper backdrop (best for contour definition). Two bulky lights are set up on easels and moved depending on the shots. Many views are taken: front, left side, right side, three-quarter face, back (to see the hairstyle or previous scars behind the ears). I also get to run the emotional gamut: "grimace," the photographer says, (this shows the laxity of the vertical cords in the neck), "smile," "don't smile," "close your eyes," "open your eyes," "chin up," "chin down." And if the ugly-lens doesn't expose every pore, the lighting will.

"My lighting is harsh and penetrating," says David Price, New York's other medical photographer. "It's like being outdoors on a sunny day at 11 A.M. The only person who would look good in it is a twelve-, thirteen-, or fourteen-year-old."

There are guidelines for plastic surgery photography, but from the photos of mascara-laden and earring-decked face-lift patients I've seen at medical meetings, it appears that the rules are often broken. Jewelry and makeup are considered "visual distractions that detract from the scientific merit of the data," wrote Harvey A. Zarem, a former chief of plastic surgery at UCLA Medical School, in a treatise on before-and-after photography. Large earrings may hide natural skin folds and facial contours, key determinants of the descent of facial fat. In "after" pictures, earrings may obscure the telltale juncture of the cheek to the ear—a seam that should look seamless. Getting women to pose naked would be easier than parting many of them from their adornments. "Some women haven't taken off their necklaces in twenty years," says Wayne Pearson, the current proprietor of the Don Allen Studio.

But the worst offense, and the biggest temptation for the photographer, according to Zarem, doesn't involve the before pictures. It's the desire to make the post-op photos "look better." It's easy enough with "photo fibbing," a term coined by *Longevity* magazine. Noses can be made smaller—visually—by using a wide-angle lens for the before view and a telephoto lens for the after, says Zarem, calling it "forthright dishonesty." Indeed, with makeup, lighting tricks, retouching, and electronic editing, it is possible for unscrupulous surgeons to simply play art director and make a person look improved in a photo without even operating on them. There are also services that supply "start-up packs" of before-and-after pictures "to jump-start the careers of neophytes."

I know of one doctor, just starting out in California, who borrowed before and after pictures of noses from a colleague. At least one patient was sold on the doctor because of the pictures. Unfortunately, he couldn't deliver the result the pictures promised. Obviously, never choose a doctor solely on the basis of a portfolio.

Doctors can't use your pictures as sales or teaching aids without your permission. My doctor will use my pictures to diagnose my problems, design the changes, and assess the results. I've ordered an extra set for my scrapbook and that's where they'll stay.

Most doctors want you to come back for "after" pictures in six months or a year. Make the arrangement yourself if the doctor's office doesn't call to remind you. As years go by, you will want those pictures to judge the staying power of the surgery. But more than reminders of the way you were, such pictures can serve as an insurance policy for both patient and doctor. The pictures can help resolve disputes if you feel you haven't got-ten enough benefit from surgery. Very occasionally a patient does look virtually the same, and the surgeon may offer a touch-up at no cost. But, more often, the patient has forgotten what she looked like beforehand.

Computer imaging in the doctor's office is beginning to replace the two-step before-and-after pictures with a three-step process I call "before-hopefully (as in, hopefully, you'll look like this when we're finished)-and-after." There is nothing as seductive as seeing your own face being morphed, electronically, from tired to fresh. Imaging can show you how you'd look if the effects of gravity were reversed. The computer can lift the brow, raise the cheek pads, straighten the nose and tilt it, and clean up the jawline.

The problem with imaging is that there is an implied promise that what can be done on the computer screen can be replicated with a knife or laser. That may not be possible.

At medical meetings, I've seen many "afters" that don't come close to the computer-imaging projection, the "hopefully" picture. On the other hand, imaging has its benefits, the chief one being that it offers a way to have a dialogue with your doctor—you can demonstrate what you want and discuss the possibility of achieving it.

A few weeks before my scheduled surgery date for my second lift, I meet with Dr. Z to look at the results of my photo session and finalize the details of my surgery. This is the last exit before the tollbooth. I will either plunk down the balance of the fee—or back out. Dr. Z breezes in with an envelope full of pictures and spreads them out on the examining-room counter. I am stunned. I feel like I am in an episode of the *Twilight Zone* and I have had my pictures taken by a camera that can see twenty years into the future.

Attractiveness is fleeting, Lakoff and Scherr pointed out in *Face Value*. We all know it will diminish in time, "through no misdeed of [our] own," along with the power that goes with it. "And like a witch's curse in a fairy tale, the loss is particularly terrifying because one never knows when it will strike, whether, indeed, it has already struck."

When it struck Madame Julie de Recamier (painted at her peak in 1800 by Jacques-Louis David on a sofa that came to be named for her), "she smashed a statue of herself because it evoked memories of her faded beauty too painful to bear."

I can empathize with the violent impulse.

Any doubts that I am a good candidate for the brow-lift are dispelled by the pictures. Let's be blunt. The vertical glabella crease between my eyebrows looks like a crack in the Grand Canyon. If that were the only problem it could be treated with a simpler procedure. But, in addition, my brow is slipping down on the bridge of my nose like sloppy ankle socks. The nose has grown hawkish. The upper lip lines have returned— as expected. The upper face is now out of harmony with the lower face.

I want the curse removed.

Almost as an afterthought, I ask, "Should we give a tug to the old lift?" My photos showed the lower face looked considerably better than before the first lift, but there was some downward descent of cheek fat. As doctors remind us, a face-lift doesn't stop the clock, it just sets it back and then it starts forward again. I could hear the ticking. I would never have thought about having another face-lift, but as long as I was having everything else. . . . You can see where this conversation was going. Dr. Z said the warranty had not expired and offered to reinforce the old lift. I like a craftsman who stands behind his work.

On the Road

Some friends were surprised I wasn't curious to try another surgeon, as if each feature needed a different name-brand designer. But I was comfortable with my choice. He did well by me the first time. Why switch? But many women feel the Astroturf is greener elsewhere. Before committing they wonder, Maybe I should be going to that guy in Brazil. Or the other one in Tahiti. Or they've heard Costa Rica is hot. What about that doctor in Florida who pays airfare down and back? Or the clinic in Tortola? Or the other one in the Cayman Islands? Affluent New Yorkers may fly to L.A. or Toronto or Dallas. L.A. women on a budget might hop down to Tiajuana (where fees are lower in part because malpractice suits are almost unknown and patients, accordingly, have no recourse if anything goes wrong), while the wealthier ones check in in New York and Honolulu. And the big-D crowd may go to San Francisco or New York. I've heard that one famous New York anchorperson went to Phoenix and another went to Vancouver. But then a V.I.P. Washington wife came to New York. With all the zigging and zagging nowadays, you can feel unadventurous for having surgery in your hometown.

In some ways it makes sense: We travel to spas—why not travel for a face-lift? "I got a chin implant and frequent flyer miles, too," crowed one woman. The patients who travel have plenty of reasons for doing it: for better prices; for secrecy; for their chance at the doctor they've heard is the Best in the World. They may consider it more glamorous, a lark, or one-upmanship. It's fine to travel for the best care, but today, with excellent doctors in every part of the country, you simply shouldn't have to travel that far to find a good doctor. And, whatever your reason, don't plan on long-distance surgery before considering the consequences and the costs. Don't underestimate the anxiety, fear, and loneliness you may feel going out of town for this operation—especially if you are alone in less-than-luxurious circumstances.

You can't do a face-lift turnaround trip in a long weekend. Most surgeons want you to stay nearby until your stitches are out—and that can take about ten days. Your surgeon will help you arrange the details. In New York, Lyden Gardens and the Carlyle and Mark Hotels have become plastic surgery hideouts. Patients are sent to these hotels with private nurses. In Los Angeles there are three or four recovery houses (don't call them nursing homes, although that's what they are) dedicated to cosmetic surgery recovery.

But remember: there's a downside to being out of town. If you are one of the few who develops postoperative bleeding or an infection, a longer stay would be required and that could wipe out any savings you might have realized by making the trip in the first place. Some doctors have reciprocal arrangements for follow-up care with colleagues in other cities, but the local doctor may resent being asked to do damage control. Even uneventful recoveries can make you wish you were home in your own bed. The postoperative period can be taxing. Many face-lift patients are surprised to find that they don't enjoy the immediate aftermath—the temporary numbness, the tightness in the neck, the sleeping propped up, the scabs in the hair, and the distortion in the mirror. Pain is rarely a problem, as that can be controlled with drugs. But the pain killers, coupled with a less-than-lovely face in the mirror and the growing impatience for "it" to be over, can cause depression. In most cases, you're able to travel in ten days, and can go out in public in two weeks, but the full effects of your surgery will evolve over a three- to six-month period. While you're in the swollen stage, it's comforting to be able to drop by your doctor's office for reassurance. The out-of-town patient can't clutch that security blanket.

Personally, I like the idea of being operated on near home. And as you'll see in chapter eight, I made more post-op visits to my doctor this time around than I did the first time. I was glad for the convenience.

Dr. Z's office has coordinated the timing of my sinus surgery with my otolaryngologist. I had hoped to get this behind me sooner, it's not easy finding a day at the end of the summer when two busy doctors are in town and have openings on their operating schedules. With the date they've chosen, I'll have less days to recover before I have to go out in public, but I have no choice. I okay a brow lift, nose nip, secondary facelift, and lip peel, and write a check for the balance of the surgical fee. The wheels are in motion. My surgery is scheduled.

Anticipation

For most patients at this stage, there are still details to decide. Will the operation be done in an office or a hospital? What kind of anesthesia, general or local? Should I trust my girl friend's advice or my doctor's on vitamin supplements?

I've got my surgery date and my information packet *and* a lot more concerns than I had the first time around, because after five years of studying this subject, I know more than I care to about what can go wrong. I have just completed an article on aesthetic-surgery complications, inspired by the death of Adrienne Brown, the wife of singer James

Brown, who succumbed in Los Angeles, two days after extensive face and body work. Ironically, the article is scheduled to appear the month I have my surgery. For reasons that make sense only to those of us who feel misrepresented by our faces, I am willing to take the risk. In fact, I feel a certain urgency. A friend is recovering from an aneurysm, which could have been fatal. Instead of that making me cautious, I want to have the surgery sooner, not later.

I remember now what I said a week after my first face-lift: "If I only had a month to live after having the lift, it would have been worth it." I also said, "If I had known what a breeze this was, I would have had my nose done."

I'm apprehensive, but not enough to back out. Just enough to be cautious. A certain amount of fear is protective. It serves as a brake on those who would book operations impulsively. Every decision for elective surgery involves a risk/reward calculation. It's no different from driving or flying or smoking or drinking. How badly do I want it or need it? What are the risks?

Scheduling surgery is not the same as ordering a new sofa, waiting for delivery, and hoping you like it when it arrives. Your actions in the waiting period can affect the outcome.

When I was considering lift number one, an experienced friend advised: "Once you make your decision to have surgery, don't schedule it so far ahead that you have too much time to worry." Good advice, but not always possible to follow. You may have to wait for your vacation time or for the surgeon. Or till you've saved enough money or arranged financing.

A reasonable waiting period, a month or two, gives you a chance to back out if you're seriously conflicted about your decision. Many doctors insist on seeing an aesthetic surgery patient once more after the initial consultation to give the patient time to reconsider. Unless you wait till the last week to change your mind, you'll get most of your deposit back. If you do go ahead with surgery, the waiting period allows you to prepare mentally and physically—lose a few pounds, for example, have your medical checkups, take a skin regimen seriously.

If you're having nose or brow surgery and you wear eyeglasses, for example, you'll want to make sure you have lightweight eyeglass frames that don't touch the bridge of your nose, because it can be sensitive for months. But don't go overboard on new frames before surgery. What flatters your face before surgery may not look great afterward (as I was to find).

I call the pre-operative limbo the *uh-oh* stage. Almost everything you read or hear seems to apply to you—and alarms you.

Time reports that being kept warm is crucial during surgery, when "Body temperature tends to plummet, which can, cause arteries to constrict and blood pressure to soar." This, in turn, can cause heart attacks. It's also known that the blood clots better when one is warm. And shivering, the body's reaction to being cold, consumes three times the normal amount of oxygen, and therefore slows healing of the skin that's been separated from its blood supply during surgery. Uh-oh!

A headline tells of a Brazilian model who nearly died from an allergy to anesthesia. Uh-oh!

Your girlfriend recommends Arnica, an herbal remedy, for faster healing. But it's not mentioned in your surgeon's instructions. Uh-oh!

Instead of stewing, collect the clippings and your questions in a file folder and make an appointment to go over final details with your doctor. No question is too insignificant to ask if it troubles you.

"Will I be kept warm?"

"I read that you can die from an allergy to anesthesia. What are the chances of this happening to me?"

"Do you have to break my nose to trim the tip?"

"How soon after surgery can I wear my contact lenses?"

"Will I lose any hair from the incisions?"

"Your pre-op instructions say, no hair coloring three weeks before and after surgery, but I can't wait that long. I have an important event. Can I color it sooner after surgery?

"I know you're not supposed to take aspirin, but I take it preventively, against heart attacks. Will I have a heart attack if I stop?

"Your instructions say to *stop* vitamin E for two weeks before and after surgery, but my girlfriend was told to take E. Why shouldn't I? What about Arnica? Do I use it topically or take it by mouth?

"Is your operating room as well equipped as a hospital's operating room?"

Often, the issues most confusing to patients are the ones doctors can't agree on, such as anesthesia and vitamins. But on two issues affecting patient well-being, smoking and aspirin intake, surgeons are unanimous.

Smoking constricts blood vessels and inhibits healing, making smokers prone to skin necrosis—the loss of skin around incisions. Some doctors refuse to perform elective surgery on someone who smokes. But smokers often lie about their habit—at their own risk. One doctor says that when he asks patients how many cigarettes they smoke per day, he automatically doubles or triples the answer.

At the least, smokers must abstain from the habit for two weeks before and after surgery, longer if possible. If you're a smoker, you could use the occasion to change your lifestyle, since continuing to smoke will undermine the benefits of a lift and cause pucker lines on the lips. On the flip side, nicotine withdrawal can exacerbate the normal postoperative depression.

Avoiding aspirin is also crucial to the success of your face-lift—or any operation in which blood vessels will be cut. Aspirin is a pain and fever reliever, but the very thing that makes it good for your heart make it bad for surgery: it thins the blood and, therefore, can cause bleeding after surgery. Postoperative bleeding under the skin (hematoma) is the most frequent complication of face-lifting—occurring in up to 5 percent of cases—and is often preventable. It's not always caused by aspirin. Exertion is another culprit. And a small number of patients lack a clotting factor in their blood. To detect this rare congenital problem, doctors routinely run a simple bleeding-time test.

The more frequent culprit in bleeding is one of a long list of vitamins and drugs. Acetylsalicylic, aspirin's chemical name, and other compounds that can cause bleeding are present in more than six dozen over-the-counter and prescription drugs from Alka-Seltzer to Zorprin and almost every headache remedy except Tylenol. Aspirin relieves pain for only four to six hours, but because its blood-thinning effects remain in the system much longer, the importance of avoiding it can't be stressed enough.

Still, no matter how strongly patients are warned, many of them are aspirin cheaters. You could fill a book with their excuses. "I didn't know there was aspirin in Excedrin." "I had a backache the night before surgery." "I just took one." "I read that aspirin wards off heart attacks. I take it every day. I was afraid to stop." It's important to note that, if you take aspirin preventively for your heart, abstaining for a few weeks should not cause a heart attack.

Even one aspirin can cause a vessel in the cheek to burst after surgery, resulting in a spreading hematoma—a painful and unsightly pool of blood that collects under the skin and may take six weeks to six months to clear up.

A broken blood vessel in the eyelid can be a sight-threatening medical emergency. If the blood becomes trapped behind the globe and is not drained, quickly, the pressure can cause blindness. In chapter eight, on complications, I'll tell what happened after a friend of mine unwittingly took a pain pill that contained aspirin the night before her face-lift.

It's important to get clearance from your doctor for *every* drug you are taking, including nonprescription medication and things from the health-food store. Diet pills and tranquilizers are problems too, because they can interact with anesthesia. By one doctor's estimate, 15 percent of aesthetic surgery patients are taking the antidepressant Zoloft—"and that's not just in New York," she said.

Elevated blood pressure can also cause bleeding. Even if your blood pressure is generally normal, it can be raised by postoperative coughing, pain, vomiting, and anxiety. These can be controlled during and after surgery by the anesthesiologist. More about this shortly.

There is less unanimity about the benefits and dangers of vitamins and herbs. Most doctors agree that 1000 milligrams daily of vitamin C (which promotes healing) is a good thing before and after surgery. There's a difference of opinion on the benefits and risks of vitamin K (which causes blood clotting) and vitamin E (which interferes with blood clotting and can cause bleeding). Some doctors ban one or the other of these; some recommend them. Follow your own doctor's advice. The instruction sheet I receive from my surgeon instructs me to take 1000 mg of vitamin C and to stop supplements of vitamin E for two weeks before and after surgery.

The influential girlfriend network—and its affiliated nutritionists— has recently—and let me warn you, controversially—begun beating the drums for ingesting the homeopathic remedy Arnica, a flower extract.

Rubbed on the skin or ingested, Arnica supposedly reduces bruising, which, for many women, is more of a humiliation than an annoyance—a sign that one's yin is out of sync with one's yang.

So what do we make of the yin and yang of Arnica? According to the Herbal Information Center, when Arnica is ingested, it stimulates blood circulation and can raise blood pressure, especially in the coronary arteries. The center advises against taking Arnica internally because it can "cause vomiting, weakness, increased heart rate and nervous disturbances." But try to tell that to a New-Ager.

At the urging of their patients, many doctors now tolerate or recommend the remedy. "Patients appreciate a doctor's openness to it," says Westchester, New York, plastic surgeon Daniel Morello. Still many of the doctors who do the largest volume of face-lifts in the U.S. oppose Arnica, saying they have noticed more bleeding in patients who take it.

The problem with homeopathic remedies, says Miami's James M. Stuzin (who routinely quizzes patients about what they're taking from the health-food store), is that their manufacture is unregulated, and product strength from batch to batch may be inconsistent.

The Arnica dilemma was recently discussed in *Technical Forum*, a plain-talking newsletter in which plastic surgeons share their clinical experience: "Comparative studies show that [Arnica] does not do any good," said one surgeon, "but then of course it doesn't do any harm! . . . If the patients believe that it works, then it probably does work for them."

Feelings

7:30 A.M.

I'm sitting on the flowered bedspread of my assigned bed in my semi-private room dressed in the limp calico smock that might as well have "patient" written all over it. A plastic I.D. bracelet is my only adornment. My husband is standing by his woman, but by his raised eyebrow and inadvertent shakes of his head, he's telegraphing, *What are you doing here, again?* He wants this to be my last trip down this road. But when one of our friends later asked him why he "allowed" me to do this again, he defended my right to make my own decisions about my face.

A stream of doctors and nurses bustle in and out, taking my temperature (in my ear), my blood pressure, my medical history, picking up the signed consent form.

For the umpteenth time this morning, someone with a clipboard wants to know what medications I'm allergic to. "I've already given the list to everyone but the elevator operator," I gripe, but, actually, I'm pleased with the attention to detail.

The anesthesiologist has come for our chat. He wants to know my height and weight. This is another time when any fibbing is dangerous to your health. The correct volume of anesthesia depends on one's poundage. This is also the moment when you know you're not having a facial.

Finally, someone gives me a Valium pill. I look at my husband. There should be His and Her doses. My spouse needs it more than I do.

My time has come. My chariot and driver await. I slide from the bed to the gurney for the trip to the operating room. (If the operating room—the O.R.—is in a doctor's office, as it is in many places in the U.S., you may wait your turn in a recliner listening to relaxation tapes, then walk to the O.R., before being asked to hop up on the table. But in a hospital you get the full treatment.)

J walks the last mile with me, down the hall past the nurse's station (I wave), past the rooms occupied by yesterday's surgical patients, down in the wood-paneled elevator to the entrance of the operating suite. There's nothing more to say. I left my instructions. "Remember," I joke, "I want a good obituary . . . with a photo." Vain in life, vain in death. The black humor couches a common expectation—that there'll be retribution for this indulgence.

The doors are pushed open. I'm sent off with a squeeze of the hand that says more than words could as my gurney driver rolls me through the double doors. By the time I'm wheeled into the operating room, I am in the ozone, awake only long enough to greet Dr. Z and remark on his cheerful red cap.

The big event is about to take place, and I'm going to sleep through it under general anesthesia. I'm in the wake-me-when-it's-over camp, with Dr. Z's approval. Not everyone agrees.

No aspect of cosmetic surgery is as controversial as anesthesia. I'm often asked, "If you're asleep, how do you know your doctor is doing the surgery?" That's like asking, How do you know the flight attendant isn't flying the plane? In a hospital it's a matter of record. In a private office, you don't know—and because perhaps 50 percent of cosmetic procedures are done under these circumstances, for thousands of women it's an act of faith. You have every right to ask your doctor if he or she will do the whole operation.

There's a Hollywood legend about a prominent surgeon—no longer practicing—who, as soon as the patient was asleep, turned the surgery over to an assistant. Today, many doctors state in their release that they will—or they won't—do every stitch of the operation. My doctor has given me his word. Suspicion is one of the reasons many patients fear going to sleep during surgery—but not the only reason.

Personal phobias, Aunt Eleanor's bad experience, and scary tabloid headlines all influence our anesthesia choices. It seems that everyone has some cautionary tale. I'm no exception. Bubbling up from my subconscious is the much-repeated story of the high-profile fashion editrice who was on the operating table, about to have a face-lift, when she had a heart attack. She awoke to find her heart specialist beside her bed—and no change in her face. "What are *you* doing here?" she asked him.

Madame editor's biggest regret, she confided recently, was that her episode happened *before* surgery, not after, and now, no one is willing to perform a face-lift on her.

When friends in the fashion world talk about face-lifting, someone invariably brings up that tale. It was on my mind during my consultation with Dr. Z, when I was shopping for my first lift. When I told him I was afraid of dying on the operating table, he had offered me the option of twilight sleep. "You'll be monitored all the time. You won't remember anything and you won't feel a thing."

Twilight sleep! I liked the idea when he explained that it was an intravenous sedative. I wouldn't feel pain, but I wouldn't be dead to the world. (But, as I learned, you might as well be.)

I checked into the hospital for the first lift, five years earlier, fully expecting to have twilight sleep. But when I was presented with the surgical release to sign, and was asked, once again, to confirm the procedures

I was having—face, eyes, neck—and the type of anesthesia I wanted, I changed my mind. I must have been brooding about it, because, impulsively, I said, "I really don't want to be even slightly aware of the operation—especially when he's doing my eyes. I want general anesthesia."

Now, here I was again, five years later—this time for sinus surgery plus a nose bob, brow-lift and touchup to the old lift. No discussion. I want general anesthesia. I don't want to be aware of any tugging or pulling. But I'm still nervous, and so is my family. "Are they going to give you too much anesthesia and you'll never wake up again?" asked my stepdaughter, voicing a common apprehension. Will merciful sleep become The Big Sleep?

Medicine's Lifeguards

"Every patient worries about dying from anesthesia," says L. David Silver, formerly director of quality assurance for anesthesia services at MEETH. "It's the number-one fear."

Good, I'm normal.

"The second fear," says Silver, "is losing control."

Some patients, explains Silver, "would like to stay awake and tell the surgeon what to do. If you were having heart surgery, you wouldn't be giving instructions. This is surgery, not a haircut. You don't tell the pilot on a plane what to do," says Silver. He tells patients, "You want the procedure. That's why you're here. You've chosen a doctor you trust. At some point you have to give yourself over to the doctor's care. If you're with a qualified surgeon in a reputable surgicenter, you should not be frightened of anesthesia. It is extremely safe."

The statistics improve every year. According to the American Society of Anestheiologists, there is only a one-in-250,000 to 400,000 chance of dying from anesthesia from any operation. But if the patient is healthy and the operation (like a face-lift) does not involve vital organs—heart, lungs, brain—the odds are probably considerably better.

The advent fifteen years ago of monitors such as the End Tidal CO_2 monitor to check carbon dioxide and the Pulse Oximeter to check oxygen saturation, the most critical measurement, has made today's anesthesia twenty-five times safer than in 1970, and ten times safer than in 1980.

An allergic reaction to anesthesia is exceedingly rare. When there is one, it is usually to a *local* anesthetic, not to an inhaled agent. A well-publicized case of allergy to local anesthetic was the 1996 case of the Brazilian soap opera star who went into anaphylactic shock from local anesthesia at the beginning of a liposuction procedure. She has fully recovered.

The fear of general anesthesia is a holdover from the days before the introduction of monitoring equipment, says Phoenix anesthesiologist Tom Nyberg, who specializes in cosmetic surgery cases. Before the advent of monitoring, "anesthesiologists would look at the patient and say 'Are you breathing?' " says Nyberg. "But today, anesthesia is less dangerous than walking on the sidewalk. You're more likely to be hit by a bolt of lightning in New Mexico than killed by anesthesia."

Nyberg, I was told, "has a cult following among Scottsdale's young executives." I can imagine popularity for certain surgeons, but for an anesthesiologist? Usually, patients can barely remember their names. The same week I was in Arizona getting an earful about plastic surgery from my ad hoc focus group (see chapter three), Nyberg dropped by my hotel to give me a short course in anesthesia. Fresh from the operating room in his green scrub suit and sneakers, he looked like a fugitive from E.R. on the set of *Hotel*. We talked about the anesthesiologist's role in cosmetic surgery. Nyberg doesn't see his job as putting people to sleep and out of pain. He sees his role as "making their day."

"The majority of people I put to sleep have not opted for surgery on a whim," he explains. "It's something they've thought about long and hard. They've changed their diet, gone to the gym. Surgery is the last step. They work for a living. This is a financial burden. Many of them have been pressured *not* to go ahead with it. Fifteen friends have said, 'You don't need it.' They have no misconceptions. The doctors I work with have shown them a tape of the operation. It's not pretty to watch. The patients have been advised of the risks. They want the benefits. Anesthesia can make or break the experience."

Not intending to trivialize cosmetic surgery, Nyberg says, "It should be a fun event like going to Neiman-Marcus for a makeover. Only this you can't wipe out. The whole episode is ruined if they don't like the anesthetic"—especially if they wake up nauseous.

The goals of anesthesia are to relieve pain and anxiety and to allow the surgeon to work without distraction, which often requires the patient to be asleep—or virtually asleep. This requires a combination of drugs and gases for three basic jobs: *pain numbing, anxiety control, and sleep.*

Narcotics or opioids (such as Demerol, morphine, novocaine, and lidocaine) are for pain. They bond to opioid receptors in the body, blocking or muffling pain so the brain senses less of it—the message just doesn't get through. The side effects of opioids can be nausea, respiratory depression, itching, and with an overdose, loss of consciousness.

Anxiolytics are for anxiety. Versed, for instance, is a particularly effective form of Valium that can be given intravenously. As Tom Nyberg says, "it calms the hell out of you. Makes you feel happy." It also gives you a retrograde amnesia—meaning you won't remember much when you wake up. But it is not a pain killer. It is often given on the way to the operating room.

Sedatives and gases knock you out. An intravenous drip of Propofol, a very expensive "induction agent," is used to put patients to sleep fast, then another gas is used to keep them asleep. An overdose of Propofol, however, can inhibit breathing. But it doesn't control pain. Only one drug takes away pain *and* puts someone to sleep—ketamine. And it has many side effects, including increased heart rate.

These three types of agents are combined to give the three basic levels of anesthesia (with infinite shades in between):

Local, the lightest, numbs pain.

Intravenous sedation with monitoring (also called *Monitored Anesthesia Care*, or MAC—what my doctor referred to as "twilight sleep") numbs pain, relieves anxiety, and keeps you in a half-sleep limbo where you can breathe on your own and communicate while being monitored.

General, the deepest, numbs pain, relieves anxiety, paralyzes muscles, and keeps you asleep while sophisticated machines assist your breathing and monitor vital functions. Frightening though it may sound, it is not your grandmother's general anesthesia.

For safety, and by law, depending on the state, any anesthesia that alters consciousness (meaning, anything more than pain-numbing local anesthesia) must be administered by an anesthesia professional—either an anesthesiologist, who is by definition an M.D. with four additional years of specialty training, or a certified registered nurse anesthetist (CRNA).

The United States is the only country in the Western world that allows nurses to give anesthesia. Many CRNAs are well trained and experienced, and in a hospital where cardiologists and resuscitation teams are available on a moment's notice, a CRNA (working under the supervision of an M.D. anesthesiologist) can be quite suitable.

When shopping for a doctor, ask the surgeon who will be administering your anesthesia. Especially if you are having surgery in an office, an M.D. anesthesiologist might increase your comfort—and the safety level. Although rare, most cosmetic-surgery deaths involve a cardiac problem and a board-certified anesthesiologist is best equipped to deal with untoward events.

Patients like the concept of local anesthesia because there is no loss of consciousness, and, the biggest selling point, no extra cost. That's because the surgeon administers it, saving the patient the anesthesiologist's fee (which averages about 1,500 dollars for a face-lift) or the CRNA's fee (which could be half that). During local anesthesia, the numbing agent, lidocaine or novocaine, for instance, is combined with epinephrine, to cut down bleeding, and administered with multiple injections. You're awake, breathing on your own, feeling no pain (except for those initial injections, which may not be fun). Local anesthesia is good for short procedures. It has an excellent track record, but it is not risk-free.

Excessive doses of lidocaine, for instance, can be toxic, thereby depressing breathing and causing a loss of consciousness and eventually seizures. Lidocaine toxicity has been implicated in complications and deaths recently following large-volume liposuction. It's unlikely that a patient would get lidocaine toxicity from the amount used in a face-lift, but it's not impossible. Another problem: "Every now and again," warns L.A. anesthesiologist Martin Gordon, "the local doesn't work in a spot. Then you give more local and more sedation and you end up giving more drugs than you would have with general, without the control."

No matter what local numbing substance is used, lidocaine, or the dentist's novocaine, it only treats pain. But it does nothing for anxiety. Anxiety, untreated, can cause a rise in blood pressure, increasing the chance of irregular heartbeats and the chance of hemorrhage. Even people with normally low blood pressure will probably have elevated pressure before an operation because of anxiety.

Up until ten years ago, most face-lifts were done under local, but as the operation got longer and more complex, and anesthesia became safer, doctors switched to general anesthesia or the compromise between local and general—intravenous (I.V.) sedation with monitored anesthesia care, "twilight sleep."

One step below general, this is, paradoxically, not everyone's first choice, but probably the most common anesthesia for cosmetic procedures nationwide, for several reasons: twilight sleep is cheaper for the patient; requires less equipment and fewer safety precautions and therefore is less costly for the doctor; and it doesn't have the name patients fear: "general anesthesia."

With "twilight sleep," the pain is blocked with narcotics (as in local anesthesia), and you are tranquilized with intravenous sedatives and in a half-awake, half-asleep limbo—thus the nickname. You breathe on your own. There is no breathing tube to get in the doctor's way and cause the occasional and brief sore throat after surgery. You wake up faster and with less of a hangover than with general anesthesia.

But these benefits are also its drawbacks: When you're sedated and breathing on your own without a tube to deliver oxygen to the lungs, oxygen intake must be monitored carefully. As must blood pressure, which is easier to control under general anesthesia. In addition, face-lifting requires turning the head from side to side and putting the neck in an awkward position—this may be better accomplished with the patient totally asleep. And in twilight sleep, the patient may sometimes feel a pain and need more local injected.

"The difference between the amount of sedation required to keep someone in twilight sleep, compared to the amount required to put someone *totally* asleep, is miniscule," explains anesthesiologist Nyberg, who feels general is safer. For the small benefit of not being totally "out," there is an increased risk of complications. When patients are breathing on their own, he says, "I have no control over their breathing. They can regurgitate. But if they're asleep completely"—in which case a breathing tube is used—"I'm controlling respiration. It's a much safer deal. Besides, a lot of people cannot lay on a slab for the required four or five hours without moving. The head can twitch at an inopportune time."

That's why some of the busiest face-lift surgeons are returning to general anesthesia. When patients insist they want local, L.A. plastic surgeon Lawrence Seifert explains he prefers general for "the maximum comfort of the patient and the safety of the procedure. But, these days the doctor's opinion means less to the patient than a statement in the media or of a girlfriend."

In or Out?

Whether you stay home or travel for surgery, you want to be sure you'll be operated on in a first-rate operating room, an issue patients too often take for granted. But it can't be overlooked now that only 30 percent of aesthetic procedures are performed in a hospital. The rest are done in doctors' offices (about 50 percent) or in free-standing surgicenters (20 percent)—both of which are, in much of the country, unregulated. But regulation is on its way, though it could take years to be widespread. Florida, for example, has just passed legislation paving the way for regulating out-of-hospital procedures.

Until accreditation is universal, it's up to the patient to ask for proof that the facility is up to snuff. There are three accrediting organizations for office surgery facilities (see page 218 for their names and numbers). California is the only state to have mandated office accreditation for ambulatory surgery using anything more than local anesthesia. In other states it is voluntary. Whether it is mandatory or optional—accreditation assures that the surgical facility meets standards for the various levels of anesthesia (proper ventilation systems and monitoring devices); that the doctor holds hospital privileges in a local, duly accredited hospital for the same procedure being performed within the office surgery unit; and that ethical standards and quality control are maintained.

No matter how well equipped the office operating room, many doctors prefer to operate on older patients, or someone with diabetes or a heart problem in a hospital. Since I'm over sixty, I feel safer in a hospital.

Beware of physicians who advertise or make a selling point out of the fact that all procedures will be done totally under local anesthesia in an office. Such promises could signal that the physician does not have an accredited operating facility or is not covered by malpractice insurance for the procedures done with sedation and deeper anesthesia. That means if you are nervous, you can't be given anxiolytics—sedatives or tranquilizers—such as Valium, Versed, or Atavar or sleep-inducing agents. These are all consciousness-altering drugs, which, depending on the state, may have to be administered by an anesthesia professional. It's a good idea to ask about a doctor's insurance situation and the certification of the operating facility.

It goes without saying that if you have a cardiac condition, or even a pacemaker, you'd be smart to be operated on in a hospital. (Incidentally, electric cautery, used in face-lift surgery to coagulate bleeding vessels—sends electric current through the patient's body and can inadvertently change the voltage setting of an implanted pacemaker. It's not fatal and doesn't rule out surgery, but pacemaker owners need to be monitored during operations and should have their pacemaker settings reconfirmed as soon as possible afterwards.)

Advice and Consent

But back to friends: they aren't always right—they can have biases and phobias and political agendas. Some want to push you into surgery. Others want to stop you from having it. We can learn from other people's experiences, but we can also be hobbled by their fears. My rule of thumb is not to take medical advice from friends who have panic attacks at the mention of surgery, faint at the sight of blood, or have an aversion to needles—not such uncommon conditions as you might think. I sympathize, but I have my own hangups (I fear surgery much less than I fear injections and implants of foreign substances that could cause inflammatory reactions—collagen, silicone, Gore-Tex, Plexiglas, gold threads, etc.).

Nor do I follow the lead of a more audacious friend who, in her twenties, pierced her own ears, and in her sixties, still fearless, went from one plastic surgeon to another, searching for someone willing to perform a face-lift on her despite medical contraindications. She finally found a willing surgeon and her operation turned out well, but she is a bigger risk-taker than I am.

Wherever the procedure is performed, whatever the anesthesia, there is a well-choreographed series of events. The pre-op photos are mounted near the operating table. The patient is laid out on the table and draped as members of the professional team take their places and play their roles. The scrub nurse unpacks the sterilized drapes and instruments. This team member knows which instrument the doctor wants before the doctor does. The doctor sections the patient's hair in rubber bands, but shouldn't need to cut any. Quick-acting intravenous sedation relaxes the patient's muscles and expresses her into sleep so that the surgeon can inject "the operative field"—it's not just a face anymore—with long-lasting numbing solution that will keep working after she awakens. (Before the operation ends, the "field" will be sprayed with more anesthetic so that there will be minimal pain on awakening. Anti-nausea medicine will be given intravenously. In the rare cases of patients with a history of severe nausea after general anesthesia, L.A. plastic surgeon Steven M. Hoefflin says he borrowed an idea from chemotherapy and uses a few drops of Marinol, synthetic marijuana, a tightly controlled substance, under the tongue, at the conclusion of surgery.

Once the local anesthesia is injected into the face, the surgeon scrubs once again and puts on gloves. The anesthesia people connect all the pulse, heart, and oxygen monitors, the blood pressure cuff, and insert the breathing tube. The End Tidal CO_2 monitor allows the anesthesiologist to know for certain that the breathing tube is positioned in the trachea—

eliminating one of the former dangers. Throughout the operation, the anesthesiologist is watching these various gauges and adjusting levels as needed and supplying oxygen.

In the Manhattan operating room, I am that body on that padded slab, and my head is not moving. I'm having general anesthesia, just as I did the first time. It's being administered by a board-certified anesthesiologist. As I said before: Wake me when it's over.

Six

ANATOMY OF A FACE-LIFT

"It is not everybody's good fortune to grow more graceful
and beautiful in advancing age."
—HAROLD DELF GILLIES, ENGLAND, 1934

We begin.

Every operation involving multiple procedures has a pre-arranged order. In my case, Act I is fixing my sinuses. During pre-op, I keep reminding myself that the inability to breathe properly has brought me to this operating room today. After the sinus doctor completes the internal work, the plastic surgeon takes over. The face-tightening is the first thing on Dr. Z's agenda. I still refuse to think of it as a full-fledged face-lift, even though it probably is. Minimizing the extent of your work is a small self-deception, popular with the lifted. I'm in good company. British actress Julie Christie, for instance, insists she has resisted plastic surgery—"save for a little work on her jawline." And she only did that in self-defense for a movie-promotion tour, she said. " 'It's really hard coming to America, where people who are older than you appear to be younger.' " Another minimizer is a media star who tells friends her recent face-lift wasn't that at all—"just a lower lift." Even though I'd rather not own up to it, my operation involves the whole face.

The second procedure I'm having is the nose refinement, followed by the brow. If the brow were done *before* the rhinoplasty, the considerable forehead swelling the brow-lift causes would distort the nose. The lip peel comes last. (If I were having an eye-lift rather than a brow-lift, it would probably precede the face-lift.)

My face has been injected with local anesthetic. Incision lines and topographical landmarks have been marked in purple. The general anesthesia has taken effect. Using a scalpel, Dr. Z starts on the right side. He makes the typical U-shaped incision that descends in front of the ear from the temple to the bottom of the ear lobe, then cuts round the lobe, and up behind the ear, before veering off into the hair. It sounds shocking—and it once was for me, before I began hanging around operating rooms. But I know now that no part of the body heals as well as the face.

Yesterday, a friend phoned to wish me luck. "You're brave," she said. But how brave do I have to be? I have antibiotics, sophisticated anesthesia, breathing monitors, and reliable professionals. Now, the first modern face-lift patient—ground zero in 1901—she was brave. We don't know her name or her age, but thanks to a New York plastic surgeon with a passion for history, Blair Rogers, we do know she was a Polish aristocrat. She dreamed up the operation and convinced Berlin surgeon Eugen Hollander to perform it on her—becoming, in the process, the prototypical twentieth-century elective-surgery patient in a field that has been consumer driven from day one.

I have tried many times to imagine how it all began from Rogers's translation of the matter-of-fact report left by Hollander. Queen Victoria has just died, and her passing is the death knell for stodgy Victorianism. The cult of youth is dawning. The Polish countess is probably preparing for some grand occasion—perhaps she's been invited to Prince Edward's coronation in London. Or a Romanov party. Or she's planning to have her portrait painted. But she is depressed by what she sees in the looking glass. She has tried chin straps and skin creams to no avail. The countess has an idea—why can't the sagging skin simply be cut away? She makes an appointment with the respected Dr. Hollander. A scholar of medical history, he once amputated a leg in seven minutes using neolithic saws made of bone and stone. Asking him to do a cosmetic procedure is like asking a brain surgeon to do a manicure. But the countess is determined.

She is dressed to charm: tightly corseted, fashionably coiffed, her lips stained with poppy petals. She arrives by carriage and is ushered into a professorial study lined with ancient medical books and Greek antiquities, Hollander's passion.

The doctor kisses the countess's hand. "How can I help you?" he asks. She raises the veil of her large-brimmed hat to reveal a tired face. She pushes up the skin of her forehead—maybe even grasping a fold of cheek skin between her fingers. "Look how loose it is," she says. Gazing through lashes that have been darkened with burnt matches, she says, "Herr Doctor. I have an idea. Why can't you just cut out the extra skin?" We know for a fact she brought a drawing. She opens her reticule and takes out a plan she has made of a face with ellipses drawn close to the hair line. He studies it. The idea is clever. She wants him to take darts in her face—a dressmaking concept applied to the skin. Interesting.

"I'm sure a brilliant man like you can do it," she says, appealing to his vanity. Perhaps she even adds, "If Graf von Zeppelin can get an airship off the ground, why can't you get rid of this excess skin?"

Hollander is hesitant, but because of his historical bent, he likes the idea of being an innovator—or maybe he is smitten with the lady. Describing the event years later, he blamed "feminine persuasion." Whatever the incentive, it works. Hollander takes the countess's suggestion and excises slivers of skin near her hairline and in front of the ear, and sews the skin back together for a tighter look. The anesthesia: injected cocaine.

Face-lifting would have taken off sooner if Hollander had presented his results to medical colleagues. (When today's surgeons perform a new cosmetic procedure, a press release is in the mail the next day.) But not wanting anyone to know he would agree to undertake what he deemed such trivial work, Hollander didn't claim his place in the record book for thirty-one years. By then, the mini-lift was an established technique and cosmetic procedures had become more respectable.

The next face-lift we know of was also performed without ballyhoo. In 1906, another German surgeon, Erich Lexer, used essentially the same technique as Hollander. The patient was an actress who complained that she was tired of taping up her sagging face with rubber strips. Lexer solved her problem by cutting out S-shaped swatches of skin in her forehead and in front of the ears and stitching the remaining skin back together. He, too, kept mum about it till years later.

Meanwhile, in the U.S. in 1906, Charles Conrad Miller of Chicago, our old friend from chapter two, the first American to devote himself exclusively to cosmetic surgery, was removing crescents of skin under the eye to cure eye bags and cutting out slivers from the nasal-labial folds— the smile lines. Miller declared that getting rid of deep wrinkles gave patients happiness and peace of mind.

Humorist S. J. Perelman spoofed Miller's 1907 book, *Cosmetic Surgery*, saying it was "calculated to make your scalp tingle. . . . Even the Brothers Mayo would have flinched" at the "violent surgery." But Miller had the last laugh. He predicted that, before long, the "featural-surgery" business would be "a most profitable and satisfactory specialty."

By the 1920s, the face-lift and nose-bobbing were thoroughly modern—like sunbathing and applying lipstick in public, although more clandestine. According to a recent biography, modern-art patron Peggy Guggenheim, who came into a $450,000 trust fund when her father went down on the *Titanic*, had her nose "tip-tilted . . . like a flower" in 1920 by a doctor who specialized "in making women beautiful."

World War I proved a boon to cosmetic surgery. Publicity about miracles of reconstruction on the war's wounded convinced the public that surgery could also accomplish beauty miracles.

And the war supplied non-combatant patients too. With five million combatants dead, there was an abundance of widows and a shortage of eligible men. For many single women, intent on becoming brides or supporting themselves, success depended on appearance. Patients told doctors they needed to look younger to get a job or keep a job or get a husband. A fresh face could make the difference between being a vendeuse or a lower-paying seamstress. There was an adage in the U.S.— the "prettiest girls went into shops, the cleverest into the factories, and the rest into [domestic] service."

Cosmetic surgery was not just an American phenomenon. Jacques Joseph, a Berlin surgeon who made his reputation rebuilding the visage of a soldier whose face was blown off by an artillery shell, admitted performing a face-lift on a woman whose business failed because she looked too old. (Joseph took two days to do a typical face-lift—one side of the face per day.) In 1922, Victor Frühwald, a Viennese doctor justified cutting out the deep smile lines of a twenty-nine-year-old woman by saying, "She intended to marry a man two years younger than herself."

Besides these practical advantages, the face-lift was beginning to have cachet. Beauty-advice books aimed at consumers began to include information on face-lifting, linking the operation to society women and film stars. In a forerunner of modern-day hype, a 1926 British book promised a lift could trim ten or twenty years off a face without leaving scars "and causes no pain." The procedure was as simple as "taking out the back of a loose waistcoat . . . as harmless as cutting the hair or nails," wrote the author Charles H. Willi. Even then, women lied about their face-work. "One fifty-year-old actress who promotes a face-cream," Willi wrote, attributes her "youthful appearance" to the cream, when, in fact, the actress had her "youth restored by cosmetic surgery five years ago—[it] took twenty years off her face and enabled her to continue her career."

Secrecy was advocated by the celebrity face-lifter of the period, France's Dr. Suzanne Noël. "Do it, but don't talk about it," she advised. Noël ran a thriving cosmetic-surgery salon in her office on Paris's rue Marbeuf. In her operating-room cap and apron, the plump-faced Noël looked more like a clerk in a patisserie than the "mother of cosmetic surgery," as her disciples called her. Her "petite lifting," the forerunner of today's lunchtime lift, was all the rage with patients who included the Queen of Belgium and the great actress we met in chapter three—whose name has never before been revealed in print (in this connection)—Sarah Bernhardt.

In fact it was Bernhardt who inspired Noël's interest in cosmetic surgery. In 1912, Noël was training to be a dermatologist, when she read about "a famous French actress" returning from a triumphal tour of America looking rejuvenated after an operation to lift her brow. (Noël never mentioned Bernhardt by name in her writings, but several doctors including a protégé of Noël's has confirmed that Bernhardt was the actress in question.) "Noël tried pinching the skin of her own face with her fingers in different places and in different directions to try to adjust the skin folds. She was surprised by what she was able to accomplish by merely lifting her facial skin with her fingers."

Noël eventually met Bernhardt, and the actress became one of Noël's first patients. The actress probably didn't pay because Noël routinely performed free surgery on celebrities for the publicity. Another of her celebrity patients was the flamboyant French music-hall star Cecile

Sorel. (Sorel scandalized Paris in 1933 at the premiere of the Casino de Paris by exposing her right breast. Those using binoculars could see the scar on Sorel's breast, proving that she had had a breast lift, another of Noël's specialties.)

Noël's techniques are documented in her landmark 1926 textbook, *Aesthetic Surgery: Its Social Role*, in which she described in detail how she took quarter moons of excess skin from under the eye, in front of the ears, under the chin—even from the back of the neck—to tighten it. One operation is documented, photographically, from beginning to end—from the operating-table views of leaf-shaped ellipses of skin being removed in front of the ears (the surgeon, incidentally, was not wearing gloves or a mask) to the post-op scene of the patient, a primly dressed matron, combing her hair after the operation and then in her hat, sipping coffee before leaving—without even a Band-aid.

Legend has it that one of Noël's patients arrived for a 6 P.M. surgical appointment dressed in an evening gown, and was finished with the "lifting" in time to keep an eight o'clock dinner date at an embassy. This cavalier behavior was possible because the wounds were truly only skin-deep—no more serious than sewing up a superficial cut. The cocaine anesthesia may also have helped. "Madame Miracle" once defrayed the cost of a round-the-world cruise by operating on shipmates in her cabin. A new opportunity awaits the adventuresome cruise-line official who reads this!

Case studies in Noël's 1926 textbook underscored the social necessity of cosmetic surgery: One patient was "a woman of sixty, who must support herself, but can't get a job selling luxury goods because she looks so old." Another was "a ruined woman of the world, fifty-five years old, forced to sing but can't get engagements. Eight days after surgery she has two engagements." Noël was also the first to write about the psychology of the face-lift, explaining how husbands of different nationalities had different attitudes about their wives' face-lifts. "The American . . . encourages his wife to have an operation" and is often present during it. The Englishman also encourages his wife, but is not present. French husbands "bristle" at the idea.

The effects of Noël's "timid interventions," as she called them, however, were short lasting. Her patients needed frequent touch-ups.

Going Down—the Face-lift Gets Deeper

How many years should a face-lift last, anyway? The various estimates I've heard sound like racetrack odds. Five to seven. Seven to ten. Eight to twelve.

Most plastic surgeons can dazzle their colleagues with photos of one or two exemplars—patients whose lifts have outlived expectations. But what are the averages? At one scientific meeting, Daniel Baker ventured that face-lifts done on patients forty-five to fifty-five years old should last from seven to ten years, but lifts done on women over sixty (my category) may last only five years.

Age may have less to do with the face-lift's longevity than the elasticity of the tissues. According to a recent European study, one in twenty face-lift patients, regardless of age, will have a significant relapse after only one year, due to skin and muscle tone. "I'd like to take away fifteen years with a lift," says one of the authors of the study, Paris plastic surgeon Vladimir Mitz, "but it's a battle."

And then there are changing criteria of how you want to look. In his experience, says Sherrell Aston, "once you see the result of a lift, you don't want to go back to where you were when you started. The lift raises your standards."

For decades the Holy Grail in face-lifting has been a technique that would give a long-lasting, natural-looking rejuvenation. During the first half of the century, the only advance in face-lifting was in the scope of the incision. By the 1940s, the incision was one continuous hairpin curve—not that different from the incision I am having. But no matter how extensive the incision, the only thing that got lifted until the mid-seventies was the skin.

"The skin lift is still the most common face-lift done around the world," says Dallas plastic surgeon Fritz E. Barton, Jr. "Just pull the skin up and back, trim the excess, close it off with tension, like pulling on the covers to make a bed. The problem is, skin is like taffy. When it's *over-*pulled, it will stretch back out to release the tension and that's where the sagging comes from." And then another lift is required. And another. And that's what gives face-lifts a bad name.

"The wind-tunnel look," a popular term of disparagement, "is three lifts done badly," explains Peter McKinney, a Northwestern University plastic-surgery professor.

Apologetic about lifts not lasting, individual surgeons made attempts at finding some deeper tissue that would make a better foundation. But most surgeons believed going more than skin-deep "unthinkable," says Mitz. Beneath the skin lies a mine field of nerves and muscles. "Damage the facial nerve and you impair not only appearance, but language and expression."

The skin lift worked best on people who needed it the least. The ideal candidate for a skin lift was "a good-looking, older woman who could be turned into good-looking younger woman," says San Francisco plastic surgeon Brunno Ristow. Thomas Rees's ideal patient was in her mid-forties, "on the thin side," he said, with high cheekbones, a strong chin, good skin, no "prune wrinkles, and a good head of hair to camouflage incisions"—a perfect description of the late Babe Paley, one of Rees's most illustrious patients. Paley and her society friends were the trendsetters who "made aesthetic surgery acceptable," says Rees. These women were "rich and privileged—and already damned good-looking. They didn't frown on the face-lift anymore. It became the thing to do."

Three developments modernized the face-lift and democratized it, making it an operation for everywoman, not just for the slim-faced Babe Paley or Audrey Hepburn, but also for a full-faced Roseanne—and me. The deeper, longer-lasting lift was at hand. But with it came increased risks, making advanced surgical training more important than ever.

The first development came in a 1974 publication. Törd Skoog, an innovative Swedish plastic surgeon, reported finding the key to a longer-lasting lift. He said the sheet of tough tissue—or "superficial fascia," as Gray's Anatomy called it—that runs under the skin from the cheekbone to the neck, could be a veritable girdle for the face if the skin and muscle were pulled up together. It would be like pulling the sheet and the blanket together when making a bed, to use the bedmaking analogy again.

What made the plastic surgery establishment sit up and take notice was one amazing set of before-and-after photos. The "Skoog woman" as she came to be known, had an "absolutely beautiful result," says plastic surgeon John N. Yousif, an anatomy expert. "Was it her anatomy or Skoog's technique? Whatever it was," says Yousif, "everyone said, 'We have to use this tissue.' " Skoog's biggest impact was in Texas. First, Dallas surgeon Mark Lemmon, and then his young partner Sam T. Hamra, became evangelists for pulling the sheet and blanket together.

All that was missing was a better roadmap of the no-man's land beneath the cheek skin—especially the relationship between Skoog's tough tissue and the facial nerve. That map was soon available. A team of plastic surgery residents in training with Paul Tessier, France's leading cranio-facial surgeon, had spent a year in anatomy labs charting the relationship of the facial nerve to the tough tissue—believed to be a remnant of a muscle. Tessier rechristened the tissue the SMAS, short for superficial musculo-aponeurotic system. Although the study was undertaken to understand facial paralysis, the authors, Vladimir Mitz and Martine Peyronie, concluded in their groundbreaking paper, that the SMAS "may be helpful in face-lifting operations."

There was considerable skepticism when Mitz presented the findings that same year—1974—at a regional medical meeting. But when the paper was published in the respected *Plastic and Reconstructive Surgery* in 1976, the international plastic surgery community paid attention. The SMAS became the buzzword. "The day after I read about it," says Aston, "I was in the anatomy lab trying to replicate the findings."

Like tailors experimenting with a new cloth, surgeons began pulling the SMAS this way and that—together with the skin, like Skoog, and in a different direction from the skin. Soon *Vogue* touted the new longer-lasting SMAS face-lift: "Good for seven to ten years," said San Francisco plastic surgeon John Q. Owsley.

With the 1980s came the third important development in modern face-lifting—Tessier's mask-lift, a procedure that uses an even deeper layer of facial tissue, the periosteum.

To understand the different face-lifting options, you need a mental construct of the face—albeit oversimplified.

The top layer is the skin.

The second is fatty tissue, including a plump cheek pad. One of the marks of aging is the descent of the fat.

The third layer is the superficial fascia or SMAS. (The facial nerves lie under the SMAS like electrical cords under a carpet, and, in certain areas, poke through SMAS.)

The fourth layer is the web of muscles that control chewing, speaking, smiling, whistling.

The fifth layer is a tough tissue called the periosteum which is attached to the facial skeleton at the nose, under the eye on the cheekbone, and at the jaw.

Only three of these layers can be used as vehicles for lifting: the skin, the SMAS, and the periosteum. And these three layers correspond to the three basic types of lifts: the skin lift, the various SMAS lifts, and the deepest, the mask- or sub-periosteal lift.

The mask-lift was designed for a young person with a sad expression. In this procedure, the surgeon goes under that fifth layer—the periosteum—with a little spatula, lifts the five layers of tissue off the bone and yanks the pile northward a few centimeters, taking away the sad look. The mask-lift doesn't do much for sagging skin, fat, and SMAS. To fix that, a skin or SMAS lift is also necessary.

When Tessier first reported the operation, he showed before-and-afters of the "Mask-lift lady." As with Skoog, "It was the only patient he ever showed," says Yousif. "She looked fabulous, and everyone said, 'We have to use this tissue for lifting.' " Mastery required practice and that resulted in a large percentage of complications—especially nerve damage—at first.

Plastic surgeons have spent the last fifteen years developing variations on these three face-lifts and debating, not always politely, the pros and cons of each. There is no one-size-fits-all lift, and no objective rating system to judge results. I know I'll get flak for saying this but comparing techniques is almost impossible. Surgeons have tried doing different procedures on two sides of the face; they have tried comparing techniques on identical twins; they have tried using panels of experts to judge results— to no avail. "There is an ongoing debate" between those who tighten deeper levels of the face and those who do simple skin lifts, says Owsley.

Complications and recovery time can be gauged, but skin quality varies widely among patients and can affect results. Even if you could get surgeons to agree, the public can't. "A patient will come for a consultation," says Daniel Baker. She'll say, 'I saw so-and-so on television and she looks terrific. Did you do her?' Two hours later, another patient says, 'I hope you didn't do so-and-so, she looks awful.' "

When surgeons aren't sniping at one another about which level of lift is best, they're debating the other issue: whether it's best to do small procedures, incrementally, as early as needed, a position stated in Dr. Gerald Imber's book, *The Youth Corridor*; or whether, as Dallas plastic surgeon Sam Hamra says, it's best to "Do it all at once, like a house—and do it between the ages of forty-four and forty-eight. You'll never have to do it again. Well, maybe in fifteen to twenty years. I don't do bits and pieces." Hamra believes the pieces of the face sag in unison and must be repositioned in unison. His "composite lift," a soup-to-nuts five-and-a-half-hour marathon that's an outgrowth of Skoog's technique, is known to require a long recovery. But then, as many people suspect, faster recovery may mean shorter-lasting results.

Who knows what I would look like now had I started my face project fifteen or twenty years earlier? Knowing how addictive this stuff is, I suspect I might look pulled by now. But there's no point in speculating. I trust I won't have a stretched look, because during this face-lift touchup, the tension is placed, yet again, on the SMAS, not on the skin. After the SMAS is tightened and the excess discarded, the surgeon reaches inside my cheek and lifts up the pad of cheek fat that has slipped down, repositioning it on top of the SMAS, over the cheekbone, as easily as you'd put a falsie in a bra.

I'm glad my anatomical deficiencies don't call for cheek implants. I've seen some subtle improvements on the right candidates, but there is a tendency to over-augment. I totally agree with Hollywood surgeon Frank Kamer, who told me once in an interview: "It's better not to have plastic in your face unless it's truly indicated." There are sunken-cheek conditions when cheek implants (made of hard plastic) *are* indicated—but the nouveau-chic, tennis-ball cheeks cropping out lately on late-night TV guests look as if they could leave the recipient of an air kiss black and blue.

The Neck on Stage

The neck comes next. Because the neck anatomy varies a great deal from person to person, what one patient had done to her neck may not be right for her best friend. A tiny incision under the chin gives visible access to the neck cords. There are many techniques for neatening up this area. If the cords are bulging, they get laced together like a corset under the skin. If there is excess fat under the chin it can be gently trimmed away or suctioned out, a recent innovation.

Ever since the 1920s, when science discovered the calorie and a slim body began replacing the prosperously plump ideal, surgeons had been looking for a way to cure the social embarrassment of excess fat. Cutting the fat out was tried a few times with disastrous results (see page 71). Doctors also tried tunneling in and shaving, crushing, scraping, rotoring the fat. After it was loosened, it was sucked out. But the after-effects of fat-cutting was often bleeding and seromas—fluid collection.

It took a world-famous beauty with a lipoma (a collection of fat) on her back—and a doctor who wanted to please her—to develop the one-step fat-suction process that came to be known as liposuction. Its development in 1977 "was a love story," says the procedure's pioneer, French surgeon Yves-Gérard Illouz, nicknamed "the king of fat."

"A pretty girl, very famous, a movie actress"—when I proposed the name of France's most enduring film beauty, Dr. Illouz said, "You're very clever"—"had a lipoma on her back. She said, 'I cannot wear a décolleté. Can you do something for me?'

"I said, 'There will be a scar.' She said, 'No scar!'

"Most people heal well on the face," he explains, but on other parts of the body, scarring is unpredictable. "One morning," continues Illouz, in a voice made raspy from years of smoking cigarillos, "I am taking a bath, I jump out of the tub. Why not suck the fat out? Every surgeon has a suction machine. We suck liquid all the time—blood, drainage. But how to suck solid tissue? I tell her, 'I will try. I will make a tiny incision, but if I don't succeed I will have to make a larger incision.'

"She says, 'I trust you.'

"So I used a sharp cannula, a tube with a sharp end" connected to his suction machine, a piece of standard medical equipment. "It was successful," he says, "although there was a lot of bleeding." While the patient didn't appreciate the historic significance of the event, she was very pleased. "She had only a tiny scar. It was a good idea," says Illouz. Over the next few years, Illouz switched to a blunt cannula and stronger suction, and Parisian women volunteered in droves to have their hips suctioned for his early studies. Word spread. And a blue-ribbon committee of fourteen extremely skeptical U.S. plastic surgeons was dispatched to Paris to check out Illouz and his technique. They came, they saw, he conquered. The technique was for body sculpting, but Illouz soon advocated judicious liposuctioning of the chin and jowls during face-lifting to restore a youthful look.

It wasn't a hard sell. Even those who believe they have earned their facial wrinkles and plan to keep them, disavow the fat under their chins. "This chin runs in my family," says a thirty-year-old designer with a blossoming TV career. She plans to have her turkey gobbler vacuumed out soon.

The tiny cannula is inserted in the sub-mental (under-chin) slit and some pink-tinged fat is suctioned out. After the internal work is done, the SMAS tightened by whatever techniques the doctor favors, the cheek pad repositioned, the vessels cauterized to stop bleeding, and some long-lasting anesthetic sprayed under the skin, the face-lift's final phase involves re-draping the skin, trimming away the excess and closing up the incisions.

Apparently patients are of two minds about how tight they want their lifts to be. Some patients "can't be pulled tight enough," says Joseph G. McCarthy, a Manhattan plastic surgeon. "You have to put a gun to their head to [convince them otherwise]. I prefer the patient who says 'I'll come back in five years. Don't make it too tight.' "

In more conservative Boston, "Don't make me too tight" is the most common request. According to Boston plastic surgeon Joel Feldman, "That's what they always say, citing three or four movie stars who have a pulled look." For many years, says Feldman, "I did what they asked. And then six months later, the patient is back saying, 'I wish I'd kept my mouth shut.' The skin stretches back. You need to look a little tight right off the bat, and then the look goes away."

Test Drives

If you can't bear the idea that the remains of countless men and women have been dissected to make your face-lift safer and more effective, you might want to skip the following.

Woe to the surgeon who isn't a good anatomist. You don't have to understand the internal combustion engine to buy a car or know anything about anatomy to undergo a face-lift, but I was curious. The technical aspects of face-lifting are so daunting to understand, I had hoped that visiting an anatomy lab would help me put "a face" on the science.

Vladimir Mitz had once offered me a tour of France's sanctum sanctorum of anatomical research, the Université de Paris Faculté de Médecine, where the SMAS research was originally done. When passing through Paris, three summers ago, I took him up on his invitation.

There is nothing like a visit to a way station for the dead to focus the mind. I can still remember every detail of that day down to what I was wearing. It was mid-July. I arrived from New York early in the morning and checked into my hotel. My first stop was Yves Saint Laurent's haute-couture show, another kind of elevated cutting. What better way to start this out-of-the-ordinary day than watching a procession of beauties modeling gowns more costly than Park Avenue face-lifts. It was a reminder of the astonishing power of youth and beauty. Beauty is riveting.

But I had other faces on my mind that day. I was to meet Mitz at a hospital at 2 P.M. When I arrived, I was handed a scrub suit and told he was waiting for me in the operating room where he was performing *live* surgery. (Because he was tied up doing a face-lift, he had arranged for others to accompany me to the Left Bank and give me the tour of the lab.) "Welcome to the real haute couture," says Mitz from behind his surgical mask.

All surgical training requires practicing on cadavers. Facial dissection, in particular, requires fresh bodies—no more than a few days old, because tissues of the face collapse when preserved in formaldehyde. In Paris, the destination for bodies that have been willed to science (and for unclaimed ones) is the Faculté de Médecine, located on a side street, two blocks from the Left Bank's Café Flore. The facade of the building is adorned with bas-reliefs depicting great moments and institutions in anatomy, including Herophilus' first dissection in the third century B.C., when, for a brief period, research was allowed on human bodies, and Ptolemy's school of zoology. Lab security is tight because body snatchers are a problem, worldwide.

Anyone who thinks a face-lift is just a cosmetic procedure sobers up fast in the eerily quiet, spotless halls of the anatomy department. The cheerful cracked yellow tile walls belie the work carried out here. No dissections are underway today, because it is a holiday in Paris. But bodies keep arriving. A door at the end of the hall leads to an immaculate preparation room, divided by curtains, where three fresh cadavers on rolling carts are being "prepared"—hosed off and X-rayed—by strapping women wearing rubber aprons and gloves. My guides and I keep a deferential distance.

"We have respect for the body," says one of them, Patrick Knipper, a plastic surgeon and anatomy teacher who, by the way, plans for his own body to become one of these cadavers upon his death. His area of study is the platysma of the neck—a muscle which in horses is used to flick flies away. In humans, it runs from the chest, up the neck, to the jaw where it thins out and becomes what we now call the SMAS. As we age, the platysma muscles relax and form those bulging vertical cords in the neck that are a stigma of aging. In the more sophisticated face-lifts, the platysma is tightened to give a smoother line.

"When we do anatomy work [on a cadaver body part], we are only given a number," says Knipper. "The name is known only to the registrar. We go into the big refrigerator in the basement. It is like a church. It's cold. No one speaks. There are many different body parts. You say to the person in charge, 'I like this one.' You put the head on a large tray on a rolling cart. You cover it with a cloth. We take it on the special elevator. If I am taking my 'body' to X ray, I look to see if anyone is coming—out of respect."

Does he find the work ghoulish? "When I work on a head, I become a technician," he explains. "There is no place for emotion. I am interested in the nerve I am researching, the plane. I have a philosophic point of view. A good physician is without sensibility during the procedure. If I have to operate on you, I have to be very precise. If I am emotional, I don't do a very good operation." But, once, Knipper admits, when he saw a body of a woman arriving, his feelings did intrude. "She still had her slippers on. In one instant, these shoes, for me, were very sad."

Most of the bodies given to science are male. But due to their dissimilar metabolism and hormones, "men and women are different under the skin," says Knipper. "The nerves are in the same place, but the underlying amount of subcutaneous fat is thinner in women"—something that has to be taken into account when transposing research experience to work on live patients.

As I write this, I recall Knipper asking me if I had ever had any plastic surgery, myself. I told him I had had a face-lift and was considering having a rhinoplasty. He tried to talk me out of it. But my other tour guide, Dr. Nora Le Go, agreed that my nose could be improved. Perhaps my nose was on my mind for longer than I want to remember.

A Millimeter Is Worth a Thousand Words

Ostensibly, Operation Upper Face (my second lift) started when I saw a candid picture of myself, in profile, a year before. I hadn't seen myself from the side in years. Was it my imagination or had my nose grown?

"Noses don't grow, but gravity pulls them down," says Jack Gunter, a Texas plastic surgeon and nose aficionado. "Everything in the face heads south of the border as we age. The amount of drop varies with skin elasticity and nose type. The hook nose tends to drop faster than the straight nose," and the drooping causes one to look stern or mean—a feature that makes older people unappealing.

It's become fairly common during a face-lift, for those over fifty to have a tiny tip lift (or upward "rotation," in surgical jargon).

"You want a slight tilt," says Gunter. "It's younger." Miraculously, when a touch of cartilage is removed from the tip and the hump is rasped down, the skin shrinks to fit like 501 jeans.

Five years ago, if you had said tip rotation to me, I'd have thought it had something to do with gratuities. But after seeing hundreds of before-and-after nose pictures at medical meetings, I realized what a difference a tiny refinement could make. Why not?

Of course, surgery doesn't guarantee improvement. It may invite gratuitous insults. The *New York Post*'s Page Six took a swipe at Jennifer Grey's new nose, saying the *Dirty Dancing* star "wrecked her movie career when she had her handsome nose bobbed."

My nose was neither here nor there—neither large enough to be considered noble, like Grey's, nor svelte enough to be elegant. Never overly fond of it, I accepted it. When I was in my teens, I knew other girls who had their noses fixed. But, pointing out my imperfection in an offhand way, my mother said, "They can only fix long noses, not wide ones." I put it out of my mind—or so I thought—until a few years ago when I submitted my face to computer imaging, first in the office of a Parisian plastic surgeon I was interviewing, and later at a medical meeting.

Seeing your image morphed on a screen is undeniably seductive. Evidence of this can be found at surgical conventions, where the crowds are thick around the imaging exhibits. I doubt that all those onlookers are shopping for equipment. Many are just curious about what they'd look like with their faces rearranged.

There's a certain auto-eroticism to the process; you are the artist and the subject all at the same time. Make that longer, shorter, thinner, rounder—tilt the nose, pull up the cheek, smooth out that furrow. Higher, lower. That's it. Perfect. Ummm. Yes. A light bulb flashes over your head. Anatomy isn't destiny. It's just a rough sketch waiting to be completed. Some elements you can revise yourself, with effort—posture, weight. Others can be fixed with a scalpel. No big deal.

Intellectually, I know that a surgeon can't always replicate the idealized image on the screen. But once you've played "What if?" and seen the possibilities, it's hard not to be intrigued.

Neither the French nose surgeon nor the computer imagers at conventions would give me a print-out of my computer metamorphosis. So, using my own copying machine, I made two enlargements of the photo of my profile, and, using a magic marker on one of them, straightened my nose with a marking pen. I mailed this makeshift "before-and-after" to Dr. Z, who had done my original face-lift. "Can you file down the bump on my nose with an emery board? But I don't want to look cute!!!" I added, punctuating for emphasis.

Admitting this, I realize I risk being accused of narcissism, youth obsession, unrealistic expectations. I prefer to see myself as a post-modern "metamorph"—anthropologist Grant McCracken's term for a person with "an impatience and curiosity to explore the possibilities of the self. It's the nature of our culture," says McCracken, "that we will seek and use the technology at our disposal."

A message came back from Dr. Z: "Come in and we'll talk about it." When we talked, I said I wanted a nose as straight as Demi Moore's, producing a photo of her—a tactic which made me suspect, since plastic surgeons are taught to avoid patients armed with movie star photos (a sign of unrealistic expectations). For all I know, Demi's photo had been retouched.

"Yes, it's possible to straighten the nose," said Dr. Z, "but you need to shorten the tip a bit for a better angle. Yes, we can do it simultaneously with sinus surgery. No, we don't need to break your nose." And no, "You won't look cute."

The first candidates for nose jobs weren't teenagers wanting to look like Myrna Loy or pop stars wanting to look like Diana Ross. They were Assyrian kings and princes—circa 700 B.C.—who considered a strong, hooked nose a symbol of power. If nature didn't supply an authoritative enough proboscis, members of the ruling class *augmented* their noses with ivory implants.

And then there was nose restoration. The extreme vulnerability of noses in combat made nose repair and reconstruction a major concern throughout history. The Egyptians included instructions for three nose repair operations in the ancient Edwin Smith *Surgical Papyrus*.

Cutting off the nose was a time-honored punishment for various offenses including adultery in many cultures—especially in India, where operations for reconstructing severed noses date back to the sixth century B.C. Among Hindus, the local potters did the surgery. A flap of skin was lifted from the cheek or from the forehead (but not disconnected) and twisted around to fashion a nose. (The "Indian operation," as the technique is called, is still used today on most nose reconstructions. In fact, it was used to rebuild the nose of Houston pathologist Dr. Seaborn [Beck] Weathers, after he lost most of his nose to frostbite on Mt. Everest in 1996.)

By the fifteenth century, the Indian operation had made its way to Sicily. Centuries before women in miniskirts were jetting to Brazil for tummy tucks, men in tights were sailing to Sicily for nose jobs. "If you want a new nose, pay me a visit," a local poet wrote to a friend in 1442. "A Sicilian surgeon has found a way to restore lost noses."

Another technique, using a flap of pliable, non-hair-bearing skin from the arm to rebuild noses, was tried and abandoned, only to be rediscovered and perfected by Bolognese anatomist Gaspare Tagliacozzi in the brawling sixteenth century, when it was called the "Italian operation." It required taping an individual's arm to his forehead for six days. Try the pose yourself:

Raise your right arm over your head. Now rest your right palm on the top of your head and rotate your elbow so it is in front of your nose and your nose is touching your right upper arm. Imagine having your arm taped in that awkward position for six days while the flap from the biceps "takes" to the nose. (Not till it develops a blood supply can the flap be cut from the arm.) Comfortable? Now I understand the engraving of the man with his arm strapped to his head that hangs in almost every plastic surgeon's office.

Tagliacozzi's critics said his operation was cruel. But he insisted it was "bearable," not painful, and a spirit booster. And he had the patients to prove it. His clinic was a mecca for European nobles who lost their noses in street fights and duels, or from venereal disease.

The church denounced facial repairs as "meddling with the handiwork of God," but the public was fascinated with the idea. The human body was the unexplored territory of the Renaissance and anatomy lectures were the equivalent of our televised space walks. The anatomy theater in Bologna where Tagliacozzi lectured to packed houses has been restored. If you visit it, you'll recognize the statue of Tagliacozzi—he's the one holding the severed nose in his hand. Today, he is considered the father of modern plastic surgery and his motto has become the motto of the profession:

"We restore, repair and make whole those parts of the face which nature has given but which Fortune has taken away, not so much that they may delight the eye but that they may buoy up the spirit and help the mind of the afflicted."

The Nose That Launched a Million Quips

Nose self-consciousness became an issue in seventeenth-century France when the ideal nose was "well made, neither too big nor too small." Cyrano de Bergerac, the political satirist, became famous for his excessively large nose, and philosopher Blaise Pascal—perhaps self-conscious about his own prominent nose—added his two cents to the ongoing discussion of one of the most talked about noses in history: Cleopatra's. For centuries it has been maligned for its strength. Had her nose "been shorter," said Pascal, "the course of history would have been different." "If anesthesia had been around, Cleopatra would have been the Cher of her millennium," speculated one writer recently. Nose job?

It's a stretch. Cleopatra VII was born around 69 B.C. and died at age thirty-nine in 30 B.C. Anesthesia *was* "around." The Egyptians apparently used mandrake, poppy (the source of morphine), white lotus, dill, and wine. These same narcotics and sedatives were used from the beginning of time until the advent, in the mid-nineteenth century, of ether, which allowed surgeons to work with less speed and more finesse—the essence of plastic surgery.

But Cleopatra's nose and her attitude toward it are mysteries forever. No one really knows what Cleopatra VII looked like. There were no trustworthy descriptions of her face written during her lifetime. The only portraits of her made while she was alive are on ancient Roman coins—and they're not flattering by modern beauty standards. She is depicted with a prominent, hooked nose. But then, the Romans didn't have any reason to glorify her—they wanted to conquer her.

The descriptions written after her death are conflicting. Some Roman writers painted a pretty picture, calling Cleopatra, "a woman of surpassing beauty" and "striking." One pointed out that "Antony fell in love with her at first sight." But a century after her death, biographer Plutarch, the Dominick Dunne of first-century Greece, said essentially that what Cleopatra lacked in looks, she made up for in personality. Her appearance wasn't "so remarkable that none could be compared with her," said Plutarch, but she was "bewitching" and "irresistible."

But not irresistible to Octavian, who was a happily married man. After Cleopatra's forces were defeated by Octavian, it's believed, Cleopatra hoped to bewitch him. No luck. "Her beauty was unable to prevail over [Octavian's] self-control." Rather than suffer the humiliation of being paraded in Rome in manacles, Cleopatra put the asp—actually a cobra—to her breast. Would a different nose have made a difference?

Sociologist Jacque Lynn Foltyn cautions against using middle-class twentieth-century values to second-guess those of a first century B.C. goddess who thought nothing of marrying her kid brother to get power and then having him murdered. "If Cleopatra had wanted a nose job, and if it had been available for cosmetic purposes, she would certainly have been the kind of woman to have one, no matter what the pain," says Foltyn, author of *The Importance of Being Beautiful*. "People have suffered to be beautiful for thousands of years."

But Foltyn suspects Cleopatra wasn't dissatisfied with her appearance. Strong noses were probably a family trait. Cleopatra VII's grandmother was half-Syrian and half-Greek. No one knows who her mother was, but her father was Macedonian Greek. "The Semitic nose was normative," says Foltyn. "Since the Greek ideal of beauty—with its high-bridged prominent nose—was much admired in Cleopatra's time," says Foltyn, "Cleopatra would have probably liked her nose and may have even viewed it as a symbol of power."

However, throughout most of history, women who had large noses, but not the power, continued to be at the mercy of beauty ideals. In eighteenth-century England, the ideal was of "moderate size, strait and well-squared; though sometimes a little rising in the nose . . . just perceivable, may give a very graceful look to it." In Victorian England, a large nose on a woman was considered a social handicap. "There is nothing more unbecoming than "high intellectual pressure," observes a dowager in Oscar Wilde's *The Ideal Husband*. "It makes the noses of young girls so particularly large. And there is nothing so difficult to marry as a large nose; men don't like them."

But a pug nose was an embarrassment too, a sign of degeneracy in the nineteenth century, when it was discovered that syphilis caused a scooped-out deformity known as the saddle nose. As late as the 1950s, a snub nose was a sign of "undeveloped intellect." The habit of judging people by their appearance—"physiognomic reasoning," sociologist Peter Corrigan calls it—encourages face-lifts and nose jobs.

Your Nose Is Everyone's Business

Knowing how much others read into noses—power, beauty, intelligence, origins, degeneracy—it's not surprising that we want to manipulate the meanings. As soon as I announced my intentions toward my nose, the dissuasion campaign started. My step-daughter couldn't have been more upset if I had planned to stick quills through my nostrils like the Cassowary tribesmen in New Guinea. She pushed her nose up with her finger and warned, "This is how you're going to look."

Where had I seen that gesture before? Oh, yes, in Brazil, at a medical conference. I was interviewing the French cosmetic surgeon, Pierre Fournier. "The difference between the beautiful and the grotesque is only a few millimeters," he warned, pushing up the tip of his nose with the top of his pen until he looked like a pig.

My friend Sue warned me that beauty standards were changing. Stronger noses were back, i.e., the noses of Kristen Scott-Thomas, Carolyn Bessette Kennedy, Donatella Versace. Trimming my nose, she said, was like throwing away your Hush Puppies the day before Kate Moss made them fashionable again.

But fashionable is not what I have in mind. Nor ideal—whatever that is. I just wanted a trimmer version of what I already had. And it had nothing to do with denying my roots—or wanting to look like Joan Rivers's sister.

I was encouraged to learn, recently, that I'm actually the typical middle-age female nose patient as described by Philadelphia plastic surgeon James Fox. These patients, says Fox, "will not accept dramatic change." They are terrified of the " 'nose-bobbed' appearance." They want "a high, straight, 'aristocratic' " nose that gives a " 'patrician-like' profile." And they want a "reduction of a bulky nasal tip."

Less is more if you've waited as long as I have. Changing your nose radically can be psychologically traumatic. Even a tiny change that is desired can be unsettling, as I was to discover. Twenty percent of rhinoplasties have to be redone because the patient is—justifiably or not—dissatisfied. A face-lift merely turns back the clock to the familiar face in your older photos. But a nose job can create a new you. The change may be desired but it takes getting used to. Even children with birth defects have a hard time adjusting to longed-for surgical improvements.

Santa Barbara plastic surgeon Jack Sheen is one of the best-known nose surgeons in the U.S. One of his patients, he says, went through a "terrible period of adjustment" when he had the hump removed from his nose. "I thought he was going to commit suicide. So I offered to put the hump back. When he knew he could get it back, he wasn't so upset."

Dissatisfied nose patients—especially men who have their noses changed in middle age—can also be dangerous to their surgeons. Many surgeons have been threatened with violence by postoperative nose patients, and at least four surgeons have been murdered by them. Perhaps Elvis Presley had the right idea. According to one biographer, when the King was considering a nose job, he previewed the effects by having buddies do it first.

I know of women who secretly crave nose surgery, but go for a consultation about their eyes, and are relieved when the doctor mentions the nose problem. But others don't appreciate unsolicited opinions. When

Stephanie, a retired ballet dancer, consulted a surgeon about a face-lift, she was taken aback when the doctor asked bluntly, "And what are we going to do about your nose?"

"Nothing," answered Stephanie, before leaving to find another doctor.

Back in the operating room, my face-lift has been completed and the rhinoplasty has begun. It's being done endo-nasally—inside the nose, so there will be no visible scars. The cartilage is being trimmed, the tip rotated, and the "rising" in my nose smoothed down with a surgical rasp. These techniques were pioneered and taught by German surgeon Jacques Joseph, the surgeon who did one side of the face per day. Joseph is now regarded as another one of the fathers of modern plastic surgery. He is present in spirit at every modern nose operation.

In 1898, Joseph thought he had found a way to make "conspicuous noses inconspicuous," without a scar. If he hadn't been a snob about speaking and reading English, he might have known that two Americans, John Roe of Rochester, New York, and Robert Fulton Weir, a New Yorker, had been using the scarless technique for ten years. Roe was the first to talk about relieving the embarrassment of having an overly prominent feature. Weir was the first to identify what we would now call the Michael Jackson syndrome, the perfectionistic patient who is never satisfied.

But if Joseph wasn't the first, he was certainly the most influential nose surgeon, credited with refining and popularizing the technique. The rich and royal of every nationality flocked to his Berlin clinic, although he also treated the less wealthy. A maharajah with a twisted nose paid through it, but a scrub woman paid nothing.

By the end of World War I, European and American surgeons, interested in the new field of aesthetic surgery, paid 100 dollars admission—a sizable sum then—to observe Joseph operating. Joseph berated his servants for serving dinner without their white gloves, but he himself performed surgery without gloves and only sterile caps on certain fingers so that he could have better dexterity. The instruments Joseph developed for nose surgery had his name etched on them and are still produced today. The chin and nose implants he designed and had made in ivory are still in use, replicated in Silastic, a hard, medical-grade silicone.

Joseph divided his cosmetic surgery patients into four psychological types, which prove as insightful as any horoscope.

Type One: subnormal aesthetic sensibility. A severe deformity may not bother them very much. They're happy with even a slight improvement.

Type Two: Normal aesthetic sensibility. They can evaluate their deformities objectively and are grateful to be free of them.

Type Three: Above-normal aesthetic sensibility. Extremely unhappy at the slightest defect. Very fussy patients.

Type Four: Pathological sensibility. People with beautiful or normal features who have imagined deformities. Sometimes can be made happy with an insignificant or sham operation.

Naturally I think I'm Type Two, but I know a lot of Type Threes.

With the rise of Hitler, more and more German patients, with so-called Semitic noses, wanted nose surgery to conceal their ethnic identity. Joseph, a Jew himself, performed these surgeries for free. But even his worldwide renown could not protect him from the Nazi juggernaut. In 1934, the Nazis began stripping him of his titles and privileges. One day, Joseph failed to show up at his clinic. Some sources say Joseph had put a gun in his mouth and shot himself.

After World War II, the nose job would become a rite of passage for thousands of young American women and men who said they wanted to be relieved of the "conspicuousness" of their noses, but were accused of wanting to erase their ethnic identity. The debate set off by Dorothy Parker when she accused Fanny Brice of "cutting off her nose to spite her race," still rages. Whether you're changing your nose to assimilate or to conform to beauty standards, or just be a better version of yourself, someone will object.

It is an inescapable fact: As long as there is even subtle racial discrimination and beauty discrimination, there will be a demand for nose jobs and it will be impossible to tease apart the motivations. For whatever the reason, the nose is simply the most prominent part of a person's face and therefore subject to the most scrutiny.

The Windows to the Soul

Festoons on Christmas trees may be very Martha Stewart, but festoons under eyes are considered very Martha Washington. During my second lift, I'm not having my eyes done—I did that during my first face-lift. But if I were having them done, they would be next on the agenda. The entry level "job" for facial-surgery patients is a blepharoplasty or eyelid lift. If, as Honolulu plastic surgeon Robert Flowers, an eye expert, says, "The eyes are the nexus of beauty," puffiness, extra skin, and fat pouches over and under the eyes detract from that beauty. (Eye fat can't be dieted away.) Many women "buy time"—putting off a full-fledged face-lift by having an early blepharoplasty. Early lid laxity, occurring at age twenty or thirty, is usually genetic. (And women who have it are quick to tell you, "These droopy eyes run in my family." "Don't blame me," they seem to be saying.)

In women, the descent of eyelid tissue can also be caused by estrogen, the same hormone that prepares the uterus to expand in pregnancy and causes stretch marks. Estrogen can loosen connective tissue, stretch lower lids and drag down eye ligaments. The eye-lift is the number-one facial procedure in cosmetic surgery. In 1997, more than 159,000 patients underwent two-lid or four-lid blepharoplasties in the U.S.

Until the 1950s, the only thing removed from eyes was skin. The current technique, removing or repositioning fat, was developed in Hollywood, the town that gave us "Bette Davis eyes." While doing an anatomy study, plastic surgeon Salvador Castenares (now retired) made the discovery that everyone had three pockets of fat in the lower lid and two in the upper. His paper on the anatomy of the eyelids—a virtual roadmap for eye-lifting—was published in 1951 and electrified the still slightly disreputable field of aesthetic surgery.

With Castanares's chart of eyelid compartments, surgeons began removing not only skin, but fat, from eyes—in the process, sometimes causing a new problem, the hollow-eye look, caused by too little fat. No matter. Castanares's blepharoplasty has become the standard: A crescent of skin taken out of the upper lid (with the incision in the fold) takes care of excess skin, crepiness, puffiness, and lid ptosis (the medical term for droop). And another crescent of skin removed from the lower lid, along with the excision of excess fat (with an incision close to the lashes) remedies the bulging bags and the deep circles which make a larger and larger under-eye drape as we age.

Except for some bruising, which can be covered with makeup, the recovery takes only about a week. And the scars are somewhere between small and invisible. The surgeon's judgment about how much tissue to remove, though, is everything. Take out too much skin, and the upper lid won't shut and the lower lid could pull down, exposing the white of the eye—a condition called ectropion. It's becoming more and more common for patients with eye problems—and those who fear them—to have a different specialist, an oculo-plastic surgeon, perform their eye-lift during a face-lift operation or subsequently.

The action, and the controversy, in cosmetic eye surgery today is in the treatment of the *lower* lid. Transconjunctival blepharoplasty, or "TC-bleph" as the surgeons have nicknamed it, is an operation for the younger patient whose eyes aren't wrinkled, but is disposed through heredity to baggy lower lids. Using an incision *inside* the lower lid, the bulging fat is removed or redistributed and no stitches are needed. Recovery takes but a few days. If necessary, the under-eye skin can be resurfaced with a laser or acid to smooth out fine wrinkles—although a peel will leave the skin red for up to three months.

But the patient who is fifty-five to sixty and has spent time in the sun—"That patient needs a traditional lower-lid blepharoplasty," says James Carraway, a Norfolk, Virginia, plastic surgeon, known for fixing eye surgery complications.

Some doctors are touting the *laser* blepharoplasty. This is a TC-bleph, but rather than using a scalpel, a light beam is the cutting instrument. There is vocal disagreement about whether a carbon dioxide laser (not to be confused with the laser used in cataract surgery) should be used to cut inside the eyelid. Personally, I don't want a laser cutting tool anywhere near my eyes, even though the eyeballs are supposedly shielded with corneal protectors. And I have company. "I don't think the laser has any place in eyelid surgery," said Thomas Baker, a pioneering face-lift surgeon in Miami. "Its best use is in the supermarket, for reading price codes."

Since the advent of the laser-bleph, there have been four cases of punctured eyeballs reported (and the doctors involved were not all novices). Advocates of laser cutting say, arguably, that the laser-cut incision heals faster. But for the day or two advantage, I'll skip it. Buyer beware.

A third option in lower eyelids is the canthopexy, which literally sews an eye tendon to the bone in order to lift the outer corner of the eye and restore the youthful tilt. "The downward tilt is terribly sad," says Flowers, who swears by this technique. "Most classic beauties like Sophia Loren and Gina Lollobrigida have a natural upward tilt." It's an exotic look that can be easily overdone.

Whatever the technique and whatever the cutting tool, the chief *aesthetic* danger in eye surgery is removing too much fat. As we age we lose fat in the face and develop a hollow look. The only way to get back the fat that was tossed away is to have fat injections. And this can be tricky business.

A bleph doesn't count as cosmetic surgery if it has to be done because the eye folds are obscuring your vision. As early as 1583 in Saxony, doctors figured out a cure for this condition. They clamped the excess skin together in a Rube Goldberg device which caused the skin fold to atrophy and fall off.

A common psychological aftermath of a "bleph" is postoperative amnesia about it and total denial. One prominent woman who is dismissive of cosmetic surgery, publicly, has had two eye jobs. She is not being devious. Like many bleph patients, she has simply forgotten. A facelift may be "condoned cheating" (as one writer put it) but a blepharoplasty is maintenance, like having a tooth filled or a precancerous mole removed. Who keeps track of every visit to the dentist? I admit, I had a traditional blepharoplasty in 1994 and it doesn't need repeating.

Many women believe they need an eye job when what they really need is a brow-lift. Only professional photos and consultations with specialists can sort out what's causing the upper eye to droop. There are even modified brow-lifts that can be done through an upper eyelid incision. As with everything in plastic surgery, customizing is the key.

A New Wrinkle in the Brow

But back to the operating room. After my nose surgery comes the brow-lift. Four-and-a-half years ago, when I was in this operating room for "face, neck, and eyes," as my invoice called it, I wasn't ready—physically or mentally—for a brow-lift. I had misgivings about a coronal lift, the technique that requires a scar over the top of the head from ear to ear.

The scar is concealed in the hair, but, as I mentioned earlier, I had heard too many reports about coronal lifts causing general dissatisfaction: a surprised look, serious hair loss around the incision, and nerve sensitivity in the scalp that can make combing one's hair an ordeal. Unless a special horseshoe-shaped incision is used, it can also make an already high hairline higher.

"I'd rather do less than more," I told Dr. Z at the time, and so my brow stayed *au naturel*. But half a decade later, my vertical frown lines are making me look chronically pained, and though I may be overdramatizing, the wrinkle forming where my brow meets the bridge of my nose reminds me of socks bunching around the ankles. I find myself holding up my eyebrows to compensate—a common indication for a brow-lift—and routinely wearing dark glasses indoors.

Doctors can't agree on brow-lifts. Some don't like them at all. Some prefer the coronal in all cases. It is the operation of choice when there is a lot of excess forehead skin that can't be expected to shrink. There is one benefit of having waited to do the brow. While my brow was on the slow downhill slide, a new way to lift it has been devised. It's called the endoscopic brow-lift.

Performing the so-called "endo brow" is like operating with chopsticks under the bed covers. This requires only three or five tiny slits in the scalp—and two long probes. On the end of one probe there's a camera (the endoscope), and a little retractor, and a light that's as brilliant as a Klieg light. This is inserted through one slit, enabling the surgeon to watch on a video monitor what he's doing with the dissector attached at the end of the other probe and inserted in another slit.

The brow tissue is lifted off the bone quite easily and repositioned upward and fixed in place with absorbable sutures (what I'm having) or tiny titanium screws that are removed two weeks later, after the tissues have attached themselves in the new lifted position. No skin is cut away, so there's no headband scar, and no resulting scalp tension, the main cause of hair loss.

But wait a minute, you say. By stretching out the wrinkles in the forehead, the skin envelope is now larger than the surface it's covering. Where does the extra skin go if it isn't cut away as it is in the coronal brow lift? Will the excess skin create a pompadour effect? Believe it or not, if the surplus isn't excessive, it will shrink to fit the skull within three to eight weeks. This is the same skin-shrinking phenomenon that occurs when a nose is bobbed.

There is increasing evidence that the brow raised endoscopically will stay put in the raised position. And a majority of plastic surgeons are switching to it. I took the word of my surgeon that he was having good results, and added the endo-brow to my surgery list.

Incidentally, while the surgeon is working under the brow, he or she can also remove or partially disable the frown muscles. I am, typically, most bothered by the deep vertical glabella crease. Some doctors remove the procerus and corrugator muscle that cause the crease, but Dr. Z believes total removal leaves an unsightly dimpling so he excises a portion of both the procerus and the corrugator muscle, allowing animation without the pained look. It shouldn't make a person look spacey, like an extra in *Invasion of the Body Snatchers*. After all, young adults without crevasse-like frown lines still manage to express concern, don't they? ("No one ever says, 'I'm sorry I got rid of it,' " says Gerald Imber.)

The first few weeks after surgery, the brow may seem as stiff as a starched collar. But expression soon returns, along with much fainter frown lines. The beauty of the procedure is that there is no long scar.

Avoiding Scarface

While you're having a lift, any growths on your face that don't qualify in your mind as "beauty marks" can be removed. Some women are emotionally attached to small moles. I'm not, and in a moment of inspired bravery before my first face-lift, I had asked my doctor, almost as an afterthought, to get rid of two tiny bumps on my face. I believed so firmly that I would have a terrible scar if they were removed that, not once, in all my consultations and preparations had I asked about the possibility of removing them. To my amazement, when they were gone, there were no scars in their place.

It is often assumed that the tendency among people of color to scar badly keeps them from having cosmetic surgery, especially face-lifts. According to the American Society for Aesthetic Plastic Surgery, only 6 percent of cosmetic surgery patients were Hispanic, 4 percent African Americans, and 4 percent Asian. But these groups are also less likely to show signs of aging, says Beverly Hills plastic surgeon Norman Leaf. "Black skin, dark Mediterranean, and Asian skin are thicker and hold up better with age than does fair Scandinavian and Anglo-Saxon skin. Darker skin may sag with time," he says, "but due to its thickness and strength, it is stronger. It doesn't form lines and wrinkles and tends to age more gracefully."

"It's a point of pride with black women that their skin ages well," says Teri Agins, a senior special writer at *The Wall Street Journal*, covering fashion. "The reason we don't have more cosmetic surgery is not because we can't afford it, because many of us can," she said. "And it's not that we don't want to look good—we do. We spend a lot of money on our hair and clothes. But when the sisters get together and dish, we certainly don't talk about face-lifts or cosmetic surgery. We wrinkle later, if at all. It's the melanin in our skin. We have a saying—it's *very* common: 'Black don't crack.'"

Agins, who is forty-four, saw the truth of this expression when she and two black classmates returned to Wellesley in 1985 for their tenth class reunion. The junior student at the reception desk couldn't believe the three were from the class of '75. "You look as young as my classmates," the student told them. At the twentieth reunion in 1995, says Agins, the difference in aging between the still-youthful-looking trio and their white classmates—who now had developed crows' feet and deepening smile lines—was evident. "Everyone told us, 'You guys look like you did when you were in college.'"

It's ironic, says Agins: "The pigmentation of our skin is the source of racism, but there's pride in the fact that it doesn't wrinkle. Having face-lifts, eye jobs—these are things we don't think we have to do. And those who do them," Agins adds conspiratorially, dropping the names of a few black beauty icons, "don't talk about it."

She also acknowledges the fear of keloid scars, something that worries patients of all colors.

If you have a fear of scars, here are a few basic facts to remember. Scarring is unpredictable but the face heals better than any other area of the body. Tension on the skin is often responsible for large scars. Smoking and steroid use complicate healing. Plastic surgeons and those trained in microsurgery can give you a finer scar. There are two categories of bad scars: hypertrophic and keloid. A hypertrophic scar is a thick, raised scar that is confined to the area of the incision. A keloid is an overgrowth of tissue, made up of excess collagen. It often has a cauliflower type of appearance that expands beyond the original scar site.

It is extremely rare for a Caucasian to heal with a keloid. They are more common in blacks, Hindus, and Malayans. According to one study, 6 to 16 percent in African populations heal with keloids, but even in this group, it is almost unheard of to have a keloid scar on an eyelid. But Leaf adds, "The face and eyes are more forgiving. People who might form keloids on the body have no problem on the face." The healing of pierced ears is predictive of face-lift scarring. If, after your ears are pierced, you have a scar the size of an olive, you are a keloid healer.

Face-lift candidates are often confused about the position of scars, fearing they'll cut across the cheeks like dueling scars on a Prussian officer. But the only visible face-lift incision is the two-inch stretch that hugs the joint between the cheek and the ear. If there is no undue tension, that area heals so well, the scar is invisible within months.

One of the most hotly debated issues in face-lifting, believe it or not, is the half-inch section of this scar that falls in front of the tragus, the scallop of cartilage at the entrance to the ear canal. Curving the face-lift incision around the edge of the tragus (post-tragal) is considered a couture touch—like turning up the hem of a designer dress and not pressing it. But on occasion—either from poor technique, excess tension, or because

ANATOMY OF A FACE-LIFT

the tragus is prominent—the "seam" on the edge distorts the tragus and pulls it forward, opening the ear up like a trumpet, which is a very unattractive look.

Some people, especially older women, have a natural gully in front of the tragus, and some very fine surgeons believe in hiding the incision in this gully (pre-tragal), where it becomes virtually invisible.

There is a growing trend, however, to treat the pre-tragal incision with contempt and make "a marketing point" out of the post-tragal incision, says Thomas Rees. West Coast doctors, in particular, use the post-tragal incision as proof of their supremacy. It takes too long for East Coast doctors to be bothered with, say the West Coast contenders.

"That's ridiculous," says New York surgeon Alan Matarasso, who says he does one-third of his cases with the incision in the front of the ear, and not to save time. The post-tragal only takes five minutes more."

There are pros and cons to both incisions. Anyone with a hearing problem should think twice about a post-tragal incision, because it can distort the ear canal and affect the fitting of hearing aids. I have a natural gully, and the pre-tragal incision I've had for both my lifts is virtually invisible—although it was red at first after each operation.

Thanks for Noticing

I'm going to jump ahead here to tell you a scar story. Much to my embarrassment, one evening eight weeks after my second lift—my nose, brow, and face-lift—my scars would be the subject of conversation.

Still healing and a bit swollen, but presentable (or so I thought) I was in Dallas to cover the annual meeting of the American Society of Plastic and Reconstructive Surgeons, the organization of 5,000 board-certified plastic surgeons.

The cab driver dropped me off at an imposing house in Highland Park, the Beverly Hills of Dallas. A local surgeon who has developed what he believes is the quintessential face-lift technique had invited me home for some Texas-sized lamb chops and a career review of before-and-after slides, which he hoped would convince me once and for all that his technique is superior to that of the face-lift mafia, his good friends and arch rivals on Park Avenue and Knob Hill.

After cocktails in the doctor's gilt-edge drawing room and dinner under a Thai temple fragment on the cozy porch, we are now ensconced in the library, side by side on the coffee-colored banquette, behind the slide projector, watching twenty-three years' worth of jowls and baggy eyes—and their corrections—come and go on the portable screen.

Suddenly, in the middle of the slide show, the surgeon turns his attention away from the faces he has lifted to my face, which he hasn't. He leans in conspiratorially, with a Cheshire cat smile and claws to match, and whispers, "I can see your scars." Dr. Pygmalion himself was reminding me that I am manufactured and my seams are showing. Was he implying that *his* scars never show—not even in the first few months? I know better. All face-lift scars, no matter who does them, are somewhat visible in the early months until they fade, but they can be hidden by hair or with concealer. The lesson here is, if you're going to be sitting next to a friend with a jeweler's loupe in her eye, or a plastic surgeon with an ax to grind, grow some sideburns or spitcurls before surgery.

That night in Dallas, I realized why the promise of the so-called "non-surgical" or "scarless face-lift" is so anxiously anticipated and why we are so willing to believe that the magic laser will do the job.

Now back to the operating room.

Seven

PRESSING OUT THE WRINKLES

"It's not the age, it's the mileage."

—RAIDERS OF THE LOST ARK

A lip peel is the finishing touch on my second face-lift, because having a wrinkled lip and a smooth brow is like wearing old shoes with a new suit. I want to smooth out the pucker lines (or the whistle lines or the lipstick bleed lines—whatever you choose to call the vertical rivulets on the upper lip above the vermilion) that come from aging and smoking and the constant activity that the lips are involved in.

Peels, like furniture refinishing treatments, come in all depths. All you have to decide is whether you just want the wax stripped and the table repolished, or whether you want the finish stripped down to the raw wood, sanded, and refinished.

I want something strong enough to give me new skin, but no more traumatic than an oatmeal scrub. While that's just wishful thinking as I write this, rapid changes in technology may make it a reality by the time you read this. Still old therapies aren't necessarily bad therapies; they're still around because they've stood the test of time and doctors using them know what to expect.

So, what are my choices? Besides the old standbys, dermabrasion (mechanical abrasion) and acids such as phenol and tri-chloroacetic acid that chemically remove a layer or two of skin, there is a tempting new therapy—carbon-dioxide (CO_2) laser resurfacing, something that wasn't available the first time I was in this position. Watching wrinkles being vaporized by the beam of a CO_2 laser is like watching PacMan on a binge. Zap, Zap, Zap. The top layer of skin disappears in a puff of smoke and the wrinkles seem to evaporate before your eyes. That's the fun part. I was tempted to try it but I ultimately chose not to. The CO_2 laser seemed too good to be true when it was first introduced—and it was.

The most common problem after CO_2 laser resurfacing is that the resulting redness can linger up to six or eight months. Knowing that the Erbium, a kindler, gentler laser, is on the way, I decided to bide my time and have a trichloroacetic acid peel—TCA to insiders. TCA is, according to Webster's, "a colorless, corrosive, deliquescent (dissolvable), crystalline substance with a sharp, pungent odor; it is used as an antiseptic and astringent." Sounds perfect for furniture finishing.

This is the same kind of peel I had back in early 1992. I was warned then that it would only last a year. It actually lasted much longer, but by late 1996 I was ready for a touchup. Muscle movement has brought the lines back to the lip—like Freddie Kruger returning to Elm Street.

Oddly, I soon found myself having to defend myself for choosing TCA instead of the laser, which is all the rage. Part of its magic reputation is that somewhere in its promotion, people began referring to laser skin resurfacing as the "nonsurgical face-lift." Some women's magazines have perpetuated the idea and you will see ads in the *Yellow Pages*—that barometer of trendy medical practices—for nonsurgical face-lifts. Hope, it seems, springs eternal that we can turn back the clock with a magic wand rather than a scalpel. And as I've learned, many women believe that if a knife isn't involved in a procedure, it doesn't count as cosmetic surgery. Never mind that acid peeling has long been called chemosurgery.

A TCA peel is deceptively simple in the hands of a pro who knows how much to use. A small amount of the acid—maybe ninety cents worth—is mixed with purified water and swabbed on the lip until a frost forms; the whiter the frost, the deeper the peel. It is rinsed off and covered with something like Aquaphor, a soothing ointment, and the peeling begins. Like a bad sunburn, it gets worse before it gets better looking. Picking, sweating, and sunning are forbidden. Tears, too, can spoil the peel. Over the course of a week, a layer of skin—as thin as tissue paper—

is sloughed off. There's little postoperative pain after a face-lift (thanks to the pain killer) but the lip peel can burn for the first eight hours. After that it's just ugly. You want a doctor with a supportive staff.

If you come away with anything from this book, remember this: a face-lift won't change your skin texture or get rid of fine lines and wrinkles; and a skin peel, though it may tighten the skin, is not a substitute for a face-lift—a peel can't get rid of a double chin or heavy jowls.

What can a peel do? A full or partial peel—whether it's by laser or other means—can enhance a face-lift. It can treat problem areas and postpone a lift in young patients with damaged skin but minimal skin laxity.

To Peel or Not to Peel

I was raised in the cream-your-face school of skin care. My mother's household goddesses were Elizabeth Arden, Helena Rubinstein, and Estée Lauder. Neglecting to cream my face nightly, I was warned, was a ticket to *rides*—French for wrinkles. I could have been more diligent. I had inherited a good complexion and believed it came with a lifetime guarantee. When Manuel Noriega was referred to as "Pineapple Face," I winced and said a silent thank-you that I don't have a pitted complexion. But I never went out of my way to maintain my good skin. By the time I was aware of cosmetic dermatologists, I had committed most of the unpardonable skin sins. I don't smoke now, but I did in my twenties and thirties. I yoyo-dieted. I tanned, or tried to. (Mostly I lobstered, until I wised up one day and quit cold-turkey.)

By the 1990s, lifestyle, UV rays, gravity, and the inexorable breakdown of collagen were winning the war with my epidermis. I needed more than the cucumber facials I whipped up in my blender. The only decision was how to wipe the slate clean and start again. A face-lift can only tighten loose muscles and pull up sagging skin. It won't do anything for uneven skin color or texture—the liver spots and discolorations, the fine lines and crinkles, dents, creases, cross-hatching, that come from the gradual thinning and stretching of the epidermis (the top layer of skin) and from repetitive muscle movements, especially on the upper lip. This is where the skin peel comes in. It's the only way to repair the wear and tear because it strips the outer layer and allows a new fresh layer to form, while at the same time rebuilding the natural collagen fibers.

Not everyone wants or needs a full-face peel. For some of us, treating the under-eye area and crow's-feet and the upper lip lines, the most unsightly areas, are all that's needed. I was amazed when a dermatologist zapped away some brown spots on my face and hands with some puffs of liquid nitrogen from a spray can. But that can't help wrinkles. Perioral (lip) lines, especially, are a key aging indicator. The muscles of the mouth are in constant motion—talking, chewing, smiling, sulking, kissing, whistling, sipping, smoking. Years of simply living eventually give the upper lip the look of a well-worn drawstring bag. Lip wrinkles are so indicative of age that character actors can add years to their faces by merely accenting their natural wrinkle lines with makeup. Try it yourself with a brown eyebrow pencil on your lip lines and crow's-feet or, if you want to go all the way, on your brow creases and smile lines as well. Look at your future face and tell me you like what you see.

I first realized my whistle lines were negative attention-getters during my face-lift consultations with Drs. W, X, Y, and Z in 1991. And it was a revelation to me that the lines could be helped. Once I was aware of them, they bothered me. I began paying attention to other women's upper lips and made some snap judgments. Some women's lips looked too good, I thought, lighter and shinier than the cheeks. But the idea that it required acid or dermabrasion to get rid of the wrinkles was frightening. I had no trouble wrapping my mind around having an inch or two of skin removed from in front of my ears and fat suctioned out of my neck. I have faith in the body's miraculous ability to heal cuts and incisions. But the idea of roughing up my epidermis or swabbing it with acid set off my fight-or-flight response. To me, acid in the face sounds like the basis for a horrible tabloid headline. What acid? How much? I wanted to see some literature on this, but only one of the four doctors I consulted originally offered any.

It would be politically correct to say my reluctance to have a peel was caused by a sentimental attachment to my rhytids (the technical term for wrinkles) and express regret about letting them go. It's popular today, after all, to romanticize other people's wrinkles. One writer eulogized them as "the lines that betray how we have worried, the creases that tell how we have laughed, the furrows that signify how we have pondered." Another got choked up observing an operation to partially disable a woman's glabella muscle, the one causing the vertical creases between the eyebrows, imagining "the ghosts of the myriad worries that furled this woman's forehead flying free: there, the times she troubled over school exams; there, the long waits for loved ones who were late; there, the years of confusion or doubt."

Call me insensitive, but I'm no more sentimental about my pursed-lip lines than I am about the pounds gained on my anniversary trip to Venice. I enjoyed acquiring them but I don't have to wear them the rest of my life. My only concern is minimizing the lines with the least discomfort and risk. A makeup artist once showed me how to soften them with concealer, but a more permanent muting is what I have in mind. If you have the same goal, you want to know which therapy to choose.

The Problem Is Older Than You Think

There is some comfort in knowing that women—and men—have struggled with similar choices for 5,000 years. It remains to be seen whether the peel, by laser or other means, will be the face-lift in the future. The acid peel was most certainly the face-lift of the past. In fact, until the early 1900s, skin irritants were the only rejuvenation remedies available.

The earliest recipe for an anti-aging paste, concocted from fruit acid, was the one I mentioned earlier—the recipe for Transforming an Old Man into a Youth—found in the Edwin Smith *Surgical Papyrus*. The ancient Egyptian medical text which dates back to 3000 B.C. described this elixir's main ingredient as an obscure fruit called the "hemayet"—believed to be the herb known today as fenugreek, a member of the pea family.

Proving that hype in a bottle is as old as hope in a bottle (or, in this case, an alabaster jar), hemayet paste was touted as "a beautifier of the skin, a remover of blemishes, of all disfigurements, of all signs of age, of all weaknesses of the flesh." And was deemed "effective myriads of times."

Women eventually became the major consumers of anti-aging treatments. Fair skin was so desirable to them, they would smear their faces with everything from poisonous mercury sublimate to Lysol and rub their cheeks with stones—the precursor of dermabrasion. Another Egyptian cure for ridges and furrows was a mixture of alabaster, salt, and honey.

The Greeks treated freckles with oatmeal paste and lemon juice. And Grecian formulas for face washes and skin emollients were among the spoils of war when the Romans conquered Athens and captured its renowned beauty doctors. Soon Rome's elders, who feared narcissism would make softies of the people who built the Empire, were blaming the Greeks for Rome's love affair with beauty masks of clay and ointments made with "narcissus bulbs, Libyan barley, honey, and hartshorn." These pastes "will never turn Hecuba into Helen," warned one Roman poet.

Nero's wife, Poppaea Sabina, Empress of Rome, had such faith in milk facials—glycolic acid—she travelled with a herd of 400 she-asses. And Cleopatra is said to have bathed in red wine, which contains tannic acid.

Sixteenth-century royalty treated wrinkles with peach blossoms crushed in almond oil, a potent exfoliant. Queen Elizabeth I smoothed her forehead creases with spiced milk and ale and set the style for face enameling—spackling expression lines and wrinkles with white paint.

The common ingredient in most of these lightening, tightening, and exfoliating treatments was some sort of acid, a stronger form of which was discovered in Germany in 1834 and remains a mainstay of peeling to this day: carbolic acid. A derivative of coal tar, it is known as phenol. Its original use was as an antiseptic. After Pasteur floated his theory that microscopic germs cause infection, Joseph Lister (for whom Listerine is named) deduced that germs in the air introduced on the hands of the operating room staff were to blame for the high incidence of surgical wound infections. The way to contain germs, theorized Lister, was for surgeons and nurses to wash not only the wounds, but their hands and instruments in an antiseptic carbolic-acid solution. Although Lister's hypothesis was controversial, the more enlightened hospitals began stocking carbolic acid. This set the stage for chemosurgery, the scientific name for skin peeling.

No one knows for sure who invented the phenol peel. One story may be apocryphal, but it is said that around the 1870s, a nurse in a European hospital was reaching for a bottle of phenolic acid and accidentally spilled some on one side of her face. The hastily devised treatment, adhesive tape to cover the burn and germicidal iodithymol powder to treat the subsequent oozing, resulted in miraculously smooth and wrinkle-free skin. To balance the effect, the other side of the nurse's face was painted with phenolic acid and the treatment repeated. Thus, it's said, was the phenol peel born.

However its use came about, the medical establishment didn't embrace this type of skin treatment. Since ancient times, physicians believed that "cosmetology did not belong in medicine." It wasn't until the nineteenth-century that dermatology even became a medical specialty. While a few of the new breed of skin doctors tried phenol on freckles, warts, and acne pits, most were too busy treating congenital deformities to concern themselves with wrinkles. But if physicians wouldn't treat wrinkles, snake oil salesmen and self-taught cosmetologists were only too happy to oblige, pushing women to ingest chalk, poisonous arsenic, and mercury—and plaster themselves with all kinds of caustic agents.

By the 1880s, "skinning" (or *encorchement*, the more sophisticated French term for phenol peeling) was a thriving, unregulated business, carried out in beauty institutes, shady salons, and private homes. And it would continue that way for decades. A 1908 *Ladies Home Journal* article, written by a concerned reader, alerted women that skinning had left one girl's face "like a piece of raw beef. . . . When it is unsuccessful, the [carbolic] acid they use to 'skin' the face eats right through." Not every case was a disaster. "When the operation is successful it leaves . . . a peach-blow skin without the fuzz," reported the *Journal*.

Every time you or I go to a plastic surgeon or a dermatologist for a skin peel, we are continuing a tradition started by the first courageous women who put their faces in the hands of lay peelers—nonprofessional, self-taught, "dermatherapists." In the first half of this century, the Dark Ages of cosmetic surgery, these lay peelers flourished underground—one step ahead of the law, their names passed from one client to another. Though their work was out of the medical mainstream, they were sought out by some of the most famous faces in the world. Some physicians—dermatologists and plastic surgeons—befriended the peelers, to learn their secrets, but kept quiet about the association for fear of being censured by colleagues.

Today, with lasers fast replacing phenol in some doctor's practices, peelers may seem like a footnote to history. But the lay peelers' techniques and formulas are being acknowledged now as the foundation of modern-day skin rejuvenation and even being legitimized in medical textbooks. Studying the formulas of the lay peelers has led to the new buffered or light phenol peel. "Phenol is alive and well and making a comeback," asserts Massachusetts plastic surgeon Phillip A. Stone, who has spent several years reconstituting and testing old formulas.

Much of what I know about the lay peelers I learned from the legendary dermatherapist Arthur Gradé (pronounced Gra-day), so my information may reflect his biases. I was given his number in the early nineties when I was trying to delve into the history of plastic surgery in Hollywood. He had never given an interview before, but was toying with the idea of writing his memoirs, so he invited me to visit him at home. Walking into his house I felt like Mary Poppins drawing a picture on the sidewalk and stepping into another world—a noir film on the dark side of beauty.

There was no doorbell. I brushed the wind chimes of Gradé's Hollywood Hills bungalow in 1994, and was greeted by a contradiction in an African mu-mu. Arthur Gradé was an octogenarian with an altar boy's alabaster complexion, a hand model's unblemished forearms, black patent leather hair, and a tart taste for gossip. Some of his stories seemed beyond belief, but almost everything Arthur told me—and some of it can't be repeated because the people involved are still alive—has checked out with other sources.

Gradé had a typical Tinseltown résumé: a made-up French-sounding name (he was born Arthur Galo in Idaho) and several occupations—

dermatherapist/opera buff/unordained preacher in an obscure sect. Although he had long since given up full-time peeling by the time I met him, well-respected plastic surgeons and dermatologists were filling up his answering machine tape, entreating him to allow them to watch him work and share his secrets. He tried to tell the doctors it wasn't the formula, but the technique that gave the un-wax-museum results he was known for. They were still obsessed with his formulas.

During my visit and in many subsequent phone conversations and faxed communiqués, he took me back to the beginning of the century, when one of the first reputable salons to offer phenol peels, he said, was the John H. Woodbury Dermatological Institute in New York. It was founded by the future Woodbury soap mogul and his brother William. Ella Harris, a cosmetologist working there, took the Woodburys' formula and opened a salon in San Francisco. One of her clients was a beautiful actress, Irehne Hobson—who happened to be Arthur Gradé's aunt.

When Harris died suddenly, Hobson saw a brighter future in peeling than in emoting. "Dear, sweet aunt Irehne broke into Harris's salon, found the formula, and had it analyzed by a chemist," said Gradé. Shortly, Hobson set up shop in Hollywood, a town where a good complexion was—and still is—especially important. She advertised her peeling service with a stunning photo of herself. Lillian Russell was a Hobson client and so was silent screen star Mae Murray. Murray had so many peels, Gradé said, that "she smiled to one side."

When Gradé moved to Hollywood in 1932 and began his career as Hobson's assistant, he recalled, "I saw my aunt peeling Carole Lombard." To make ends meet, Hobson and other lay peelers supplemented their incomes by selling formulas, sometimes with the ingredient ratio altered or one ingredient missing. The peelers weren't giving much away because the real secret of success was, as Gradé had already told me, in the application technique (when to powder, when to tape, when not to tape) rather than the phenol mixture itself.

Before long, there were as many peelers as manicurists in Hollywood, most with invented European lineage. And they were all plotting to get one another's formulas and clients. "It was like the film, the *Maltese Falcon*, where they were all killing one other for the statue," Gradé said. Many a movie career was saved by a peel. Peeling, said Gradé, proved a godsend for Mae West, who was forty in 1932 when she signed with Paramount and started making films. She was desperate to look youthful.

Not that face-lifting wasn't available. It was an option then, but a frightening one because anesthesia was crude, antibiotics not yet perfected, and incisional scars more visible than they are today. In any event, a face-lift could only pull up loose skin. It couldn't do much for acne-pitted or finely wrinkled skin or skin irritated by toxic makeup—conditions magnified by photography. A good result from a peel was like airbrushing on a photo. It tightened skin and got rid of freckles, fine lines, and crow's-feet without incisions and without changing one's hairline.

But peels could be dangerous, and every once in a while a career was destroyed by one. After a peel, Richard Barthelmess, the silent screen star, described by his frequent co-star Lillian Gish as having " 'the most beautiful face of any man who ever went before the camera,' " developed a droopy eyelid and was forced to retire at forty-seven.

Bad results notwithstanding, the peelers were Hollywood's biggest beauty secret. Hobson was soon eclipsed by Jean De Desley (née Maime Elizabeth Larson). De Desley's name, in keeping with the custom among cosmeticians to give themselves a European gloss, seems to have been a variation on her husband's name—Disley. De Desley operated out of a large house on Fuller Street in West Los Angeles and, with a sly nod to her Mississippi birth, always flew the Confederate flag. Because she wore nothing but black after Rudolf Valentino died in 1926, many believed she was the legendary "Lady in Black" who visited Valentino's tomb every year on the anniversary of his death.

No one knows who taught De Desley, but her formulas became a virtual gold standard of rejuvenation, passed down from one peeler to another (including Gradé who was one of her assistants for a time) until they were finally passed along to today's leading plastic surgeons and dermatologists.

One of De Desley's students, according to a legal document given to me by Gradé, was Sarah Shaw. She went into business calling herself Antoinette La Gassé and claimed her father was a French surgeon who invented the peel during World War I—a fabrication repeated so many times, it now turns up in medical textbooks as fact.

Shaw/La Gasse's celebrity clients included Mae West and Dietrich, who patronized several peelers—a ploy that, in Gradé's opinion, ensured no one could say definitively how much work Dietrich had had done. Despite constant run-ins with the law (in California, putting anything stronger than, say, a fifty-percent strength fruit acid on someone's face is and was a felony if you don't have a medical license. Only physicians are supposed to use deep peeling agents), Shaw/La Gassé practiced peeling until her death in the early 1950s. She bequeathed her formulas to her dressmaker, Cora Galenti, who (no slouch at myth-making) later claimed they came from her Italian grandmother.

Galenti set herself up in a twenty-three-room villa on 7158 Sunset Boulevard, called the Fountain of Youth, and advertised "Permanent Rejuvenation without Surgery." She promised that her 2,500-dollar peel would take twenty to forty years off a face and claimed that Gloria Swanson, Ginger Rogers, George Raft, and, of course, Dietrich were her clients.

A November 1956 feature story in *Confidential* magazine—"New Faces for Old Without Surgery . . . The Miracle the Medicos Can't Explain"—written by Galenti's press agent, brought Galenti national attention and legal harassment. It was rumored, but never proved, that one Galenti client, an actress, killed herself over the results of a peel and that another was found in an alley, dead due to renal failure from phenol toxicity. Phenol is a potentially toxic chemical that is absorbed into the blood stream and, in sufficient quantities, can affect the heart and the kidneys if the patient isn't monitored properly during the procedure. That's why the non-physician peelers did their peeling in stages, a few square inches at a time, sometimes over the course of several days so as not to put too much phenol into the patient's system at one time.

In 1959, after paying an 1,800-dollar fine for practicing medicine without a license, Galenti relocated to Las Vegas and opened the five-bedroom Fountain of Youth Ranch. Again there was trouble. In 1961 she was arrested and convicted of postal fraud for mailing pieces that claimed her treatment involved "no burning, no peeling, no pain" . . . while erasing "sometimes forty years of sags and winkles." Testifying otherwise, one ex-patient said the treatment felt "like liquid fire."

Only one notable—Jean Parker, the actress who played one of Katharine Hepburn's sisters in the 1933 film *Little Women*—came to

Galenti's defense. After being sentenced to ten years in federal prison, Galenti fled to Mexico City, where she ran a mail-order face-cream business, returning to L.A. in 1993 to die at age ninety-five. Her son still operates the mail-order operation.

Galenti's saga was the inspiration for *Faces*, the 1991 novel by *Vogue*'s former beauty editor, Shirley Lord—a tale about a woman disfigured by a face peel. Such stories contributed to the fear of phenol peels.

Lana, Marlene, and Grace

Arthur Gradé, who used De Desley's system, was the peeler's peeler, but his price—up to $12,000 for a full face peel in recent years—and his attitude alienated many. Gradé wouldn't take a patient he didn't like. Paulette Goddard and Liberace passed his scrutiny. So did Swanson, who Gradé claimed he peeled for *Sunset Boulevard*, and Constance Bennett, whom he worked on for *Madame X*. "I inherited Dietrich from another peeler," said Gradé. "She was quite difficult. Extremely nervous. She only ate one meal a day. . . . When she was older, no one wanted to peel her."

Gradé also claimed he was recruited to peel Howard Hughes, who wanted the treatment but was afraid of it. Gradé recounted how a complete laboratory was set up in a warehouse in an industrial neighborhood, and over a period of three years, under the supervision of Hughes's physicians, Gradé demonstrated his technique on four stand-ins. "I don't know if I ever peeled Hughes himself or just some doubles," said Gradé.

He also claimed a Hollywood agent arranged for him to go to Monaco—to peel Princess Grace—in the late sixties. "They sent a private plane for me. I had my own room in the palace. There were five doctors supervising, giving the sedation. I felt like a cuckoo who came out on the hour to swab on the peel solution. It was so secretive, I wasn't even allowed to go to a restaurant. The prince was away. I spent seventeen days there. The princess ended up with a pink, glowy face."

It was, however, hard not to be skeptical when Gradé claimed, "I gave Pope Pius XII an angelic look. He was into every rejuvenation therapy."

In fact, it is well known that the pope underwent a course of rejuvenating sheep-cell therapy in 1954 with the Swiss physician Paul Niehans—a cure that was popular with such luminaries as W. Somerset Maugham, Bernard Baruch, Gloria Swanson, and Charlie Chaplin. In that context, a skin peel for the pope wouldn't have been totally out of the question.

Working without monitoring equipment or deep sedation, the lay peelers stayed out of trouble, as we know, by painting on the acid, a small patch at a time. It would take Gradé one full day to paint the face, section by section, with rest periods in between. "It was like painting the White House with a tiny brush," says a surgeon familiar with the technique. The second day the face was covered with special tape. After forty-eight hours, the tape mask came off and powder was applied. Ointments and compresses were applied on subsequent days. Gradé wanted to control every aspect of the recovery. He allowed his clients only herbal teas and inspected the contents of their purses, tossing out vitamins that would interfere with healing. "Even lip pomade can ruin the results," he said.

Gradé's phenol peel took twenty-one days in all. Lana Turner, he said, had a nurse drive her back and forth to his house every day for three weeks. On seeing the finished effect, she exclaimed, "No more sins." In a thank-you note typed on flowered stationery and dated May 25, 1977, Turner thanks Gradé for past kindnesses and tells him he is more than "just a face rejuvenator." "It sounds like a monologue from one her movies," noted Gradé, "but it meant a lot to me at the time."

> Dear Arthur . . . Because of you I am a more self-confident person and feel so good about myself. Going through the process isn't an easy experience, but when you are through you feel like you have not only had your face peeled away, but your soul also. . . . Lots of love—Lana

In 1970, *Coronet* magazine anointed Venner Kelsen " 'the Tiffany of lady face-peelers.' Whenever an actress tested a little 'tired' for her upcoming picture," said *Coronet*, "she was simply sent to Venner Kelsen." Kelsen was a formidable woman with a Kewpie doll face and curls that matched her French poodle's. She pretended to be Swedish but she was born Edna Kelsey in the U.S. She also claimed she learned peeling in Europe, but she really learned it from Madame De Desley and Arthur Gradé.

Kelsen's face creams and electric facials, her bread-and-butter business, were all the rage with clients as diverse as Helen Gurley Brown and Louis B. Mayer. Brown plugged Kelsen's services in *Sex and the Single Girl* and in *Cosmopolitan*. Barbara Walters featured Kelsen's 245-dollar mail-order "Face Saving" machine on the *Today* show. But the big money for Kelsen was in the 3,000-dollar phenol peels she performed in her Beverly Hills duplex on Hollywood royalty from Merle Oberon to Gary Cooper. As one of the last links in the long chain of lay peelers, her apprentice, Jacques Thomas, who now practices in Ashland, Oregon, has been called on, of late, to speak at medical conventions about peeling.

The biggest problem for the peelers was pain control. Theoretically, they could not administer narcotic pain medication. Some peelers brought in doctors to give shots to the patients. "Kelsen's pain treatment was nonchalant," says Thomas. "When she peeled my face, without any sedative, it was the most excruciating pain I'd felt in my life. I felt like I was on fire. Some people don't need anything for pain. Others have zero pain tolerance. Venner suggested that her patients get something from their doctor in advance. If they didn't, she had a stash of outdated pain pills in a shoebox in her closet. The patient could be in the worst pain, but Venner never lost her cool."

Scarring was always a possibility. Kelsen herself had a scar on her cheek from one of her many peels. But the worst possibility was a waxy and mask-like appearance. "Some women in Beverly Hills looked like ghosts," says Thomas. "The skin was almost scar tissue. Makeup would slip off. These weren't Venner's patients. She had beautiful, natural results."

Phenol Goes Mainstream

The mainstreaming of the phenol peel began in Florida. In 1957, Miriam Maschek, a former patient of Cora Galenti, and her husband Francis opened the House of Renaissance (later changed to Derma-Lift Salon) in North Miami Beach. Peeling with acid by nonphysicians was illegal in California, but not in Florida—home to hordes of people with sun-damaged skin. Cora Galenti accused the couple of stealing her formulas. The Mascheks claimed the recipes were given to them by Antoinette La Gassé. Soon the Mascheks received national attention when a *Chicago Tribune* investigative reporter—Norma Lee Browning—who had set out to expose them, ended up praising their work in a fourteen-part 1960 series detailing the day-by-day, post-peel transformation of forty-one-year-old Chicago housewife, Anne White, who went from someone with " 'dried up, weather-beaten skin' " to " 'a butterfly, with the pink, glowing skin of a newborn.' "

The medical community was incredulous, believing the series was a "hoax." But two respected Miami plastic surgeons, Thomas Baker and Howard Gordon, became believers after seeing some of the Mascheks' patients in person. When the Mascheks refused to share their formula, Baker and Gordon began to construct it from patients' descriptions.

"All of them described the smell of carbolic acid and a tan powder that smelled like iodine," recounts Baker in the introduction to his 1998 textbook on skin resurfacing. "They reported how areas [of the face] were covered with adhesive tape." Baker began searching the dermatological literature and found physicians' formulas that dated back to 1903, but had not been published until the 1950s because of the stigma attached to treating wrinkles. He began experimenting with weak phenol formulas on rats and rabbits. The first human trial was on his own freckled forearm. Then "a small spot on the face of our brave secretary. Then the forehead of an elderly woman who was undergoing a face-lift." The results were "beautiful" and complications almost nil.

It took Baker and Gordon and a few other pioneers ten years to make science out of what was essentially folk medicine—figure out the exact ratios of phenol, test recipes, do tissue research, publish papers, and convince skeptical colleagues that phenol peeling was a legitimate therapy with extraordinarily long-lasting results, especially for middle-aged women suffering structural skin damage from too much time spent in the sun. "It took a lot of courage to apply this solution to a patient's face," said

Clyde Litton, a Washington, D.C., doctor who did some peel studies in the early sixties.

The moment of truth for the plastic surgery community came in 1972, when Baker and Gordon brought a patient who had had a full-face phenol peel to a plastic surgery society meeting in Las Vegas. More than 100 years after phenol was first used for wrinkles by lay peelers, the phenol peel was finally an accepted therapy with a dignified new name: chemosurgery.

After the Maschek's divorce, Francis married and teamed up with another Galenti alumna, Jacqueline Stallone, mother of Sylvester, who would have a colorful and controversial career in skin treatment before she became an astrologer to the stars. But phenol peeling has become so respectable now, Stallone, who says she once peeled Clara Bow, has been invited to share her secrets with plastic surgeons. She declined. And at a recent medical conference, like a food critic comparing sauce vinaigrettes, a Nevada plastic surgeon evaluated the ratios of croton oil (which increases the depth of the peel) and liquid soap (which buffers it) to phenol in the formulas of various lay peelers including Gradé, Maschek, and Kelsen.

Too bad Arthur Gradé wasn't alive to learn of his elevation in the pantheon. He departed this world in as colorful a manner as he lived in it. In the spring of 1996 Gradé told a friend, "Tomorrow I am going to meditate and light a candle. If the candle goes out, I'm going to be leaving you." The candle went out. The next day he was dead.

My Acid Trips

In 1992, I had yet to meet Arthur Gradé or know the ins and outs of skin peels, and I was at a loss deciding what to do about my upper lip wrinkles. I learned in my first consultations that I could have the doctor plane down the indentations with one of various abrasives: a metal burr, a diamond-edged brush, or sandpaper spinning at 10,000 revolutions a minute. This technique (introduced in 1905 by a German surgeon) showers the atmosphere with skin and blood—one reason it is falling out of favor.

I asked a Beverly Hills friend, a plastic surgery aficionada, for the low-down on dermabrasion. "Prepare for your lip to swell up to three times its size. The pain can be controlled, but it's uncomfortable for a week, and women get panicky that it will always look terrible. You'll have to wear sunscreen for a long time, or it can become pigmented." Instead, she suggested sending the wrinkles on a shorter vacation, swabbing them with a more dilute acid—a light peel, to be repeated once a year, as she does.

And as it turned out, a light peel was exactly what Dr. Z, the fourth plastic surgeon I consulted, suggested during my initial consultation with him. "You don't need a heavy peel or dermabrasion," said the surgeon. "A light TCA peel isn't painful. You might have to do it again in a few years, but you'll like the results." I have since learned that TCA is a less potent cousin of the phenol peel. You might call it "phenol lite." Dating back 150 years, TCA is an acid that coagulates the protein in the top layers of skin, causing them to peel like a sunburn. It is effective for mild wrinkling and it usually has to be repeated every few years. Its main advantage—it is less likely to bleach the skin (as phenol can) so it is effective for a partial face peel, say, just the lip, and poses no danger to the heart. That doesn't mean it's benign. In stronger concentrations it can cause a higher incidence of hypertrophic scarring than phenol.

The TCA peel proved to be the ugliest part of my recovery after the first lift, leaving me with a swollen, brown, then red, then pink upper lip that required expertise with concealer for a month or so, but was well worth the effort. Not having had a phenol peel or dermabrasion, I have no basis for comparison, but I like to think I chose the lesser of three evils. As predicted, I was very happy with the result, and also, as predicted, it didn't last, despite regular applications of a glycolic acid cream.

Four and a half years later, when I decided to have a brow lift, I was ready for another peel. As Los Angeles dermatologist Mark Rubin says in his *Manual of Chemical Peels*, skin aging, "is a chronic disease, like hypertension or diabetes," needing "daily treatment to control and reverse [it]." Obviously, in my case, the daily treatment needed to be stronger.

By 1996, when I am again confronted with the decision about how to treat my lip, I have, in addition to the three original choices—phenol, TCA, and dermabrasion—the option of resurfacing with a carbon dioxide laser.

The Light Fantastic

I first heard about laser resurfacing in 1995 at a plastic surgery convention in San Francisco. It was happy hour in the ballroom of the Down-
town Marriott and I was standing near the Taste-of-Chinatown table. I
was introduced to Thomas Roberts III, a North Carolina plastic surgeon,
and told he was the man of the hour. With missionary zeal, Roberts
explained how he had taken a loan to buy a 120,000-dollar laser that
would revolutionize plastic surgery. He was making a presentation the
next day, and to convince any Doubting Thomases, he had brought along
two patients in their sixties—a man and a woman—who had had their
wrinkles tightened up and smoothed out by the laser, and still looked
natural. The results seemed impressive.

By the close of the meeting, dozens of surgeons were thinking about
taking out second mortgages on their houses. I make it a policy not to do
any impulse shopping on this beat—but I confess, I was tempted when
Roberts said I'd be an ideal candidate for laser resurfacing. But I heeded
the warning of another physician who advised, "Let your best friend try
it first." I wrote an article about it instead.

Most of us may have forgotten, if we ever knew, that the word laser is
an acronym for "light amplification by stimulated emission of radiation."
This is a process that relies on a hot and powerfully destructive beam of
light. There are over 100 laser wave lengths in use in medicine, each with
its unique target. The Q-switched ruby laser removes blue and black tattoos
and liver spots. The Q-switched YAG laser destroys yellow-pigmented tattoos. The flash-lamped pulsed dye laser treats port-wine stains.

For more than twenty years, laser researchers have been trying to
develop a laser that could safely and predictably resurface healthy but
sun-damaged or aging skin. While the conventional continuous beam
CO_2 laser, invented in 1964, works well on warts and lesions, it is not
considered safe for resurfacing. Of course, that didn't stop doctors from
using it for just that purpose. There were some successes, but the risks of
severe burns weren't worth taking.

In 1990, Coherent, the world's largest laser manufacturer, produced the ultra-pulsed CO_2 laser. It did not need FDA approval because it was a modification of an existing technology. The operating principle is simple: The light is delivered in rapid bursts, like a machine gun. The dwell time—the time the pulsed light is on the skin—is so brief that, theoretically, surrounding tissue is not damaged. In 1991, San Diego dermatologist Dr. Richard Fitzpatrick was asked by Coherent to test the laser on skin lesions. When that worked well, he tried it on healthy but wrinkled skin. "The first few patients, I couldn't believe how good they looked," says Fitzpatrick, who suggested design modifications. "I wanted to be sure it wasn't a fluke."

Other doctors were enlisted to do tests in the U.S. and in Australia, where sun damage has reached epidemic proportions because of the thinning layer of ozone gas (which acts as a filter for ultra-violet rays) above the continent. "When we put an ad in the paper for volunteers, the word of mouth from previous patient/volunteers was so good," said Fitzpatrick, "we had over 350 phone calls"—ten times what was expected. The usually cautious researcher was soon predicting that laser resurfacing would be "a simple outpatient procedure, little more than having your nails done, and not as serious as having molars extracted."

Thanks to a cleverly orchestrated p.r. effort by manufacturers, the public knew about the "laser for wrinkles" before many plastic surgeons did. It was introduced to the vast daytime TV audience by Geraldo Rivera in March 1995. Beating Oprah, Phil, and Sally to the ray gun, Geraldo became the first talk-show host to have his crow's-feet (two on each side) zapped, live, on national TV. Using a 120,000-dollar machine to lase away four little lines seems like overkill, but doing anything more extensive would have required deeper anesthesia and might have forced Rivera to take time off to recuperate.

The operation looked too miraculous to be true. As the audience watched through goggles (a necessary precaution since a laser beam, bouncing off, say, a shiny button, could blind someone) the doctor/wizard aimed a swing-arm wand of light at Geraldo's crow's-feet and vaporized the offending creases. On contact with the skin there was a snap, crackle, and pop and a puff of smoke as a dot of epidermis was blasted into a fine white ash. Pop, pop, pop. Lo and behold, when the ash was wiped away, the skin underneath was as soft and pink as a baby's.

The home viewers reacted in a frenzy of desire. I want it. Where can I get it? Geraldo had to add two phone lines to handle the inquiries. And surgeons all over the country were besieged with calls from patients anxious to sign up for laser wrinkle removal.

What the audience didn't see was how many passes it takes to get rid of deeper lines, how raw the skin looks an hour after the treatment when the swelling and oozing sets in, and how long it takes for the skin to return to normal. The viewers didn't ask questions—they just accepted the treatment as a miracle.

One would think that after all the complaints, accusations, and law suits about breast implants, the public would be more skeptical. But the laser has a special connotation, says Eugene Halton, professor of sociology at Notre Dame and a popular culture specialist. "What were God's first words?" asked Halton. " 'Let there be light.' God is often identified as 'light.' "

Ronald G. Wheeland, the dermatologist whose research a decade ago paved the way for the development of pulsed-laser technology, was worried that the laser wasn't ready for prime time—let alone afternoon TV. "None of this has been submitted for peer review in medical journals."

Many people predicted the laser would eventually replace the deep phenol peel. An added advantage, the laser doesn't affect the heart. Any doctor who didn't have one of these 120,000-dollar zappers was soon feeling "like a Neanderthal." But then came the downside. Doctors whispered among themselves that there had been several cases of severe scarring from the laser—and not from inexperienced surgeons. Even more alarmingly, there had been a handful of cases of eyeball perforation. Experience soon showed that skin eruptions on the fourth or fifth post-op day often heralded a herpes infection. Hurriedly, the word went out that it would be wise to prescribe anti-herpes medication routinely before laser peels. Fungal infections were also reported but were almost impossible to diagnose because laser-ablated skin is so raw.

Doctors with a big investment in CO_2 pulse lasers began sweating. At subsequent meetings, surgeons reported that the recovery period is not easy. One study found that 20 percent of patients can count on post-operative itching. Patients who had been promised they could go back to work in two weeks found that swelling and redness lasted longer than that. "Put it in your consent forms that redness is *guaranteed* for four months," doctors were advised.

The TV show *Primetime Live* followed a woman through a full-face laser peel. She said "I probably would think very seriously before doing the laser again. The next day, said Jeff Dover, a laser dermatologist affiliated with Harvard's medical school, patients all over the country called to cancel their appointments for laserbrasion. Obviously there was a big difference between having four small crow's-feet zapped—à la Geraldo—and a whole face.

Doctors soon admitted that the zapping was the fun part. Managing the recovery was more serious business. At meetings they warned one another not to undertake laser resurfacing without having a full-time aesthetician in the office. One doctor showed a one-week post-op picture, the crusted-yellow stage he called "the Dijon-mustard face" and shared his patient-selection criterion for a laser peel: "the kind of person you'd want to take on a camping trip—she'd better be a good sport."

Even the doctors who were most rhapsodic at first have tempered their enthusiasm. "You can get spectacular results—and spectacular complications," says Roberts, the early booster. Another doctor with a large face-lift practice reported, "postoperative care is horrendous. A lot of hand-holding is required. The laser has to be better to abandon other techniques. But how much better are the results? The eyelids are spectacular at three months, but not as good at nine months." He concluded, "I'm not giving up dermabrasion."

By 1996 there were tissue studies and long-term comparisons with other peeling techniques, and the results were not what was hoped for. The magical early improvement in skin appearance, it was found, was partially due to the excessive swelling. "Everyone looks smooth as glass at two to three months, unrealistically tight, a wonderful result," reports one of the early boosters. But as the months wear on, the swelling subsides and by eight months—just when the embarrassing redness finally clears up—the wrinkles, especially the ones caused by dynamic muscle action, start returning. One study found 8 to 12 percent of patients will have a "persistence or recurrence" of lines.

Meanwhile the list of cautions was growing. A history of cold sores (herpes infection) or shingles. Anyone who has taken Accutane, the acne medication, within the previous two years or anyone who ever had radiation treatment on the face for acne or other problem—even if it was twenty years ago—could get skin necrosis from the laser. The patient with ruddy skin or who experiences a burning feeling from soap "could be your worst nightmare," says Roberts, who advises his colleagues to use a jeweler's loupe and lay hands on the faces of post-laserbrasion patients to feel for incipient hypertrophic scar formation. Scars can be headed off, he says, by weekly injections of the steroid Kenalog. But too much Kenalog and you could get skin withering.

The consent form I saw at one laser clinic warns that treatment of the skin with the CO_2 laser "is relatively new." That, as far as anybody knows, "the laser is as safe as other destructive therapies." And that "long-term side effects of laser light on human tissue are not yet completely known." There may be long-time sensitivity to sun, and even to cosmetics, it's said.

Another caution is using the laser during a face-lift on skin that has been undermined—that is, lifted and separated from its blood supply. Undermined areas, such as the outer cheeks, can't be peeled until the lift has healed and the swelling subsided.

The more I learned about CO_2 laser resurfacing, the less I wanted it for my 1996 lip peel. I admit when I first saw those two laser patients in San Francisco, I was tempted. But the more people I spoke to, the more cautious I became. I finally decided to repeat the medium-depth TCA peel. Insiders say that frequent TCA peels are the secret to the not-yet-lifted beauty of one of France's most enduring actresses—the woman in chapter six who may have been the inspiration for liposuction.

In a few years, when tissue studies are completed, the underlying mechanism of laser ablation may perhaps be fully understood and the machines improved. "Cool" lasers like the Erbium YAG are here now and show promise, although the benefits are even more short-lived. I like knowing they will be options when I need a peel again. But if you are having any laser treatment, make sure your doctor has experience with the treatment and an office staff to handle aftercare. Whatever agent is used— mechanical abrasion, an acid formulation, or laser light—remember all peels are controlled burns that slough the top layers of skin, allowing new collagen and a fresh new epidermis to develop.

A beneficial side effect of any skin peel is skin shrinkage. It may be enough tightening for a forty-year-old (who doesn't need a face-lift), but nothing that exists now can correct the loose jowls and double chins of a fifty- or sixty-year-old. To cinch up sagging muscles and re-drape stretched-out skin, you need a surgical face-lift. "Patients have to remember that aging is more than lines in the face," says Thomas Baker. "Don't forget old mother gravity. Everything in our bodies is trying to fall to the center of earth. Patients will be less afraid of the laser. But it's not going to replace face-lifting."

Fill 'er Up—or Not

Though I have yet to try them, there are other techniques now being used to combat the effects of aging on the skin. Arnold Klein, the L.A. dermatologist, likes to say, "There's a time to fill and a time to pull." Only a consultation with a dermatologist or plastic surgeon will tell you when you're ready to pull. If you're not ready, there is no shortage of fillers.

I could cushion the lip cracks and smile lines with threads of Gore-Tex, a synthetic bio-material not to be confused with ski parka fabric, or I could use the even newer SoftForm Facial Implant, another synthetic. Early uses of Gore-Tex implants have often been clunky. I've seen smile lines that look like the welting on the seams of slip covers. The nasal-labial fold deepens when fat in the cheek begins descending. During a face-lift, the cheek fat is elevated and the fold—which can't be entirely eliminated—is minimized. Theoretically, it's better to raise the fat than to fill the gully made by its descent.

I could also have tiny globules of silicone injected into the crevices, but I'd have to go to Europe for that. Liquid silicone was classified as a drug by the FDA in 1965 and reclassified as a medical device in 1976. Although it has been effective when used in minute quantities to fill out wrinkles, creases, and scars, it is not approved by the FDA for injection for any cosmetic purpose because it can migrate and cause inflammation and discoloration of surrounding tissues as well as form nodules of tissue. It is currently illegal for U.S. physicians to promote or use the injection of liquid silicone, but if you want it badly enough—and many women do— apparently, you can still find someone to supply it.

Or I could get in line for the most popular wrinkle treatment of all: bovine collagen, a temporary line plumper. (Collagen is a protein extracted from the hides, hooves, and bones of cows. Collagen Corp. says it has its own medical-grade herd, which is fed a gourmet diet. Translation: no mad-cow disease.)

If I didn't object to putting Plexiglas in my face, I could also plug the facial indentations with Artecoll, beads of Plexiglas suspended in bovine collagen from a German pharmaceutical herd. (English cows have been banned in Holland and Germany for more than ten years.) This concoction brings to mind the sawdust on the floor at my local plastics-supply house, but the manufacturer says that micro-particles of Plexiglas have been used successfully in hip and jaw implants. Soft tissue, however, responds differently to foreign substances than bones do. And that's why Artecoll is currently in research trials in the U.S. with fifty investigators, but it is not yet available on demand.

Even if your Plexiglas padding works, your wrinkle problems may not be over. An interesting side effect, noted in research on Artecoll: when you pad out a wrinkle caused by muscle activity, a "secondary" fold may develop right next to the padded one. Twin peaks and valleys.

But be advised: before treatment with pure collagen or any collagen-containing substance such as Artecoll, you have to be tested (with a patch on the arm) for collagen allergy. About 3 percent of the population is allergic to it. Ideally, testing should be done at least twice (some physicians give three tests) four to six weeks apart. Even when you appear not to be allergic, an allergy to collagen can develop during the course of treatment.

The symptoms of collagen allergy are enough to further furrow any brow: rash, hives, joint pain, headache—not to mention shock and diffi-culty breathing (very rare), as well as infections, abscesses, open sores, lumps, peeling skin, scarring, triggering of herpes simplex. Even if you're not allergic, one place I would avoid getting shots of Zyplast, the heavy collagen, is in the frown lines between the eyebrows. In two unfortunate cases, the shots were given too deeply, into a vein, causing blindness. Even a person's own fat injected into that vein, by mistake, has caused partial blindness.

Despite the small risks, at least 1 million people worldwide have tried collagen in the past two decades. Having a standing appointment for injections is as commonplace today as regular dental visits for plaque removal is for some folks. Hollywood runs on collagen. The biggest win-ners at the Academy Awards are the face-plumpers who treat the glit-terati beforehand. But Hollywood doesn't own collagen. Even Andy Warhol confessed to a once-a-month habit.

I may be one of the last holdouts. Saying no to collagen when I haven't even had a collagen-allergy test makes me sound phobic. I don't refuse flu shots, vaccinations, and inoculations. So what's my problem? You would think that someone who has had two face-lifts would be the first to try fillers. Flying back from a dermatology convention, recently, a doctor sit-ting next to me told me my attitude was generational. He said younger women want to do everything *short* of having surgery.

I'd feel that way too if I wasn't so aware of history.

It's amazing how willing we are to believe in these magic bullets. The modern quest for the ideal bio-compatible implantable filler for hollows and depressions has been going on since the beginning of the century. The history of plastic surgery has been the story of enchantment, followed by disenchantment, with one material after another. Gold, silver, porcelain, ivory, celluloid, cork, gutta-percha (the latex used in golf balls), stones from the Black Sea, and even Vaseline were used, often with disastrous results, to build up noses. Having a gold thread basted under the chin from ear to ear is a controversial technique for keeping the chin taut.

There was no FDA watchdog in the late nineteenth century when respected Viennese surgeon Robert Gersuny started filling facial hol-lows with paraffin, a coal-tar derivative. The treatment proved particularly disastrous, causing tumors, infections, and hideous disfigurement. But once this scourge was unleashed, it couldn't be contained.

Women's magazines repeatedly warned readers of the dangers of waxy injectables. In 1912, the *Ladies Home Journal* told the sad story of the girl who wanted "Sunken Cheeks Made Plump." The paraffin "formed a lump in each cheek." Another woman who had her face filled out with paraffin, the *Journal* reported, was not only "pitifully scarred," but her neck would "remain stiffened for life." Solid grease wasn't any better despite a London physician's promise that it was "no more objectionable than putting "artificial teeth in the mouth or pads in the shoulders of an evening coat."

But despite the warnings and the horror stories, some doctors persisted in offering paraffin, and women bought it. Its problems were well-publicized by the mid-1930s, when the Boston-born Gladys, the Duchess of Marlborough—considered to be the most beautiful woman in the world—had paraffin injections in her forehead. The material later slipped down inside her face to her chin, giving her a lumpy and lopsided appearance. She became a recluse until her death in 1977. Today, the duchess is a symbol of women who believe "it won't happen to me."

Silicone was the sixties' magic bullet. When astronaut Neil Armstrong walked on the moon, on July 21, 1969, he took that "one small step" in silicone boots. Those were the days—before all the breast-implant litigation and the (still unproved) allegations that silicone causes autoimmune diseases—when we wanted to believe that there was Better Living Through Chemistry. Liquid silicone was touted as "the least reactive substance for human use." When injected, it appeared to cause almost no reaction. A panel of eight prominent physicians were invited by Dow Corning to set up a test program. At the same time the FDA began studying the long-term effects of injecting liquid silicone in the body. A permit was required to use the material.

Reporting on the study in 1971, *Vogue* called liquid silicone a "sensational discovery" with great promise for plastic surgery. An injection of this "new synthetic material" could smooth out "corrugated foreheads . . . frowns congealed between the eyebrows . . . austere lines compassing the mouth." Best of all, the pubic was told, silicone shots required "no heavy anesthesia, no surgical knives, no sutures. . . . A tiny syringe half filled with a slick, clear fluid, a slender needle, and an amber-colored antiseptic . . . is all the equipment the doctor needs." Twenty drops a session, two sessions a week, and in two weeks the wrinkle would be plumped up. According to *Vogue*, "A woman could cheerfully become 'addicted' to liquid silicone."

There was only one problem. Medically purified *liquid* silicone was limited in availability due to reports of wandering clumps of silicone under the skin of the kind mentioned above after too-generous injections. Oops. Consequently, the material was being treated like a drug and tested under the watchful eye of the FDA. Only the eight physician-investigators were allowed to dispense it. There was, however, a black market in less-pure industrial silicone—which many predicted, correctly, would lead to "countless disasters."

One of the eight physician-investigators was Hollywood's star plastic surgeon of the day, Franklin Ashley, who had rebuilt Ann-Margret's face and performed Phyllis Diller's first face-lift. He favored silicone injections for the face but not as breast injections.

Another investigator, Reed Dingman, head of plastic surgery at the University of Michigan, was more skeptical, worrying that foreign materials "triggered the body's defense mechanisms, resulting in inflammatory reactions [and] infections"—a concern that was eventually borne out in a small percentage of patients. But for a brief period, at least, even Dingman was beginning to think that silicone was different—"the body *did* tolerate it."

After interviewing all eight investigators in person, *Vogue's* reporter came away optimistic that "this darling man-made chemical Schmoo won't let anybody down." The message was not lost on beauty seekers.

Jolie Gabor, mother of Zsa Zsa, Eva, and Magda, was a satisfied user and helped spread the good news about silicone. When Gabor complained to a plastic surgeon about frown lines, she recalled in her autobiography, he came at her with a needle. She protested that she was on her way to a cocktail party. " 'They won't even notice it,' " he told her, quickly giving her two injections. Gabor describes how she ran to the mirror and saw that the wrinkles had been miraculously smoothed out.

" 'It is not even red. What did you do?' " she asked. " 'Nothing,' he said calmly, putting away his instruments. 'What I gave you was silicone.' "

The treatment cost twenty-five dollars. Gabor claimed she never again had trouble with her forehead, although six years later she underwent a face-lift. Eileen Ford, owner of Ford Models, was another who has stated publicly she found silicone injections trouble-free.

For others, however, the injections were more than a letdown—they were a disaster. One of the most visible and outspoken casualties was Elaine Young, a Beverly Hills realtor and an ex-wife of the late actor Gig Young. In 1977, Young admired a friend's new high cheekbones and was told they were the result of liquid silicone injections. For the next year, once a month, Young received silicone injections that may have been impure. Three years later she noticed the shape of her face changing. The silicone was moving and hardening, she had trouble speaking and closing one eye. From then on, she endured years of cortisone shots to reduce inflammation and thirty-two corrective operations to remove the silicone—"all because I wanted to look more beautiful," she confessed. Young, who is something of a crusader, has become an emblem of the catastrophic effects of liquid silicone shots. She has given interviews to *The New York Times*, the *L.A. Times*, and *60 Minutes*, among others, warning the public of the dangers of this beauty treatment.

A 1996 report by three plastic surgeons on injectable silicone concluded that the material can cause facial nodules, cellulitis, ulceration, and migration. "While the incidence of complications may be low, when they occur they are devastating and cannot generally be resolved satisfactorily." Silicone injections were such a public health problem in Nevada, that in 1976, the State Legislature made the injection of silicone into any part of the body a felony offense. Still, I get calls from women, bemoaning the fact that they don't know where to get silicone injections anymore.

By the time you read this, three new skin fillers will be available to you that weren't to me. The first, if you don't mind the donor, is "Dermalogen"—injectable collagen made from sterilized, cadaver skin treated with anti-viral agents. Supposedly its benefit over bovine collagen is that there is very little chance of an allergic reaction. The second is also from human donors—AlloDerm® Universal Soft Tissue Graft, skin tissue (screened for the donor's medical history) from a tissue bank (FDA approval is not required).

The third is "autologous" collagen, made from one's own excess skin, discarded during surgery. It can be stored for up to six months and injected, a little at a time. Now there's an injectable I would feel extremely comfortable having under my skin. Autologous collagen can also be made by harvesting some skin from the buttocks in a small procedure that can be done under local anesthesia.

Numb and Number

If you have nothing against being injected with a detoxified form of the deadliest poison in the world, the latest line tamer and, to date, the best temporary treatment for those frown lines between the eyes is Botox, a trade name for a highly dilute form of botulinum toxin (BTX). Until the 1970s, BTX's only use was as a quick, cheap weapon of mass destruction. In germ warfare circles, BTX is called the "poor man's atomic bomb." In the war against wrinkles, it can be life-enhancing.

Ironically, if inhaled or ingested, a millionth of a gram of BTX can paralyze the lungs and cause asphyxiation. But a billionth of a gram, injected strategically in forehead frown lines, crow's-feet, or vertical neck cords, muzzles the nerves that command the muscles to contract. The muscles are immobilized, and the skin covering them flattens out.

The effects are temporary. After three or four months the muscles have to be injected again. At 350 to 1000 dollars per area, three or four times a year, the costs can add up. A mini brow lift might not cost any more than five Botox sessions.

In the 1970s, a San Francisco eye surgeon began using BTX to control eye muscle spasms. A patient in one of the trial programs noticed that her brow wrinkles relaxed after the injections. Because BTX was the first bacterial toxin to be used as a medicine, it underwent one of the strictest trials ever conducted by the FDA before being approved in 1989 for three muscular conditions. But there's no law to stop doctors from using it any way they choose, and many began using it for wrinkles.

Injecting Botox is like painting by numbing. Depending on the artistry of the doctor, patients look like airbrushed versions of themselves or wax figures out of Madame Tussaud's. There have been no cases reported of systemic reaction to the toxin. But there have been some less than beautiful results. Injections in the wrong spot or bending over within four hours can cause a drooping eyebrow. And some people have experienced visible bruising.

It says something about the desire for youthfulness that in spite of botulism toxin's reputation as "an evil microbe . . . the most poisonous poison," patients are actually lining up for "germ warfare" on their wrinkles. Indeed, the same people who would lie down in front of a bulldozer to stop a toxin-refining and -packaging facility from being built in their backyard, are begging for Botox right between the eyes. "If I drop, I'm going to look amazing," says a Miami Beach Botox user, Andy Singer. Because of Botox, she says, "I look younger at thirty-nine than I did at twenty-five."

Actually Botox has the most trouble-free safety record of any wrinkle remedy. But as its use increases so does the incidence of drooping brows.

A Simple Solution

Just because the latest "fix" is available and presumably safe doesn't mean it's for you. The treatment must fit the problem. Back in the operating room, during my second lift my between-the-eye frown line doesn't need temporary paralyzing. It has been neutered surgically. I don't want to go back for shots every four months. And Botox is not the solution for anyone's lip lines. Botox around the mouth would give a person temporary lip paralysis.

Considering how much thought went into my deciding how to treat three-square inches of upper lip area, the lip peel itself is anticlimactic. It takes about two minutes. The TCA crystals are diluted with distilled water in a small glass to the desired strength (light- or medium-depth) and swabbed on with a soft applicator till the skin forms a pink or white frost (again depending on the desired depth).

My operation is over. My head is wrapped in a gauze helmet with two drains attached to tiny incisions behind my head (to drain blood and fluid for two days).

My freshly peeled lip is being covered with Aquaphor. For the next few hours I'll be sleeping off the anesthesia in the recovery room. Someone has called my husband to tell him the operation was a success—I'm alive. For the next two weeks it's up to me to be a good patient and a good sport and not do anything to undo the results.

Having been through this before, I thought I'd breeze through it again—but I was to find the second time harder then the first due, probably, to my impatience. The real test of a doctor, and a patient, comes after the surgery and consists of the real or imagined concerns that crop up during this postoperative period. I was to have both: in particular, I *imagined* the time it took the lip to heal to be a complication rather than what it really was—an *expected* annoyance.

Eight

PARDON MY APPEARANCE; I'VE JUST HAD A RUN-IN WITH A PLASTIC SURGEON

"The pleasing punishment that women bear."
—WILLIAM SHAKESPEARE, COMEDY OF ERRORS

It's late in the afternoon, the day of the operation.

How long have I been back in this bed? I have no concept of time. It seems like dusk. I'm aware of someone applying cold compresses to my forehead. It's my nurse. I sense someone else in the room. I peek out from under the compresses and see the blurry image of my mother standing at the foot of my bed.

"Is this Joan?" she inquires tentatively. This is my first inkling that I am once again unrecognizable, something I will see for myself, later in the bathroom mirror.

I can imagine her—like Scarlett, in *Gone With the Wind*, searching the sea of wounded for Ashley—looking for her daughter among the gauze-wrapped heads on this floor. There's a dull ache in my head. The only thing I can truly feel is my lip burning. The nurse keeps greasing it with ointment.

Soon J arrives. I'm grateful he recognizes me. I remember the story told by Nola Rocco, proprietor of the Hidden Garden, an L.A. recovery house, of a husband who spent an hour holding the hand of the wrong woman.

Later, that evening, when a friend calls to find out how I'm doing, I can hear J whispering, "She's in pain."

"I'm not in pain," I protest weakly. "I just don't feel like dancing."

I'm scheduled to stay two nights with private nurses. It sounds self-indulgent, but I'm grateful to a friend who warned me the first time around. "There was no pain. Just some discomfort," she said. "I looked horrendous. You must have nurses for at least twenty-four hours to keep changing the ice packs on your eyes." She said her son and husband did that for her, and it wasn't a great idea.

I followed her instructions. As I've said before, why spend top dollar for surgery and then have a do-it-yourself recovery in the sensitive first twenty-four to forty-eight hours?

But the drive-through face-lift is becoming the norm. These days, some 75 percent of all cosmetic surgery is performed in hospital outpatient clinics or private operating rooms that may or may not have provisions for overnight stays. This means patients must scramble for after-care. In Manhattan, many patients are sent to a hotel with a private nurse. In L.A., patients often go to a special recovery house. I've heard of an arrangement in Salt Lake City where a nurse opens her own house to a patient for a week. Or you can go to *your* own home, with or without a nurse. Depending on the amount of anesthesia, the length of the operation, and the number of procedures involved in the facelift (are you having only a face- and neck-lift or the face plus nose, sinuses, eyes, brow, cheek implants, lip augmentation, and a full or partial peel?), it may be asking too much of yourself to get dressed and climb into a car or taxi a few hours after a face-lift while you're still feeling the anesthesia after-effects.

But some women find it psychologically preferable to act tough, thus downplaying the seriousness of a face-lift. If they admitted to themselves that the operation was such a big deal, they might not want to go ahead with it. Their stoicism isn't entirely an act. Many face-lift patients, according to one study, tend to be "assertive, perfectionist people . . . who need to feel in control of situations." In other words, they need permission to be dependent.

Allow me to give it to you. A face-lift *is* real surgery. In most cases, everything goes well. But in a small number of cases, problems occur.

When they do, the friend or spouse taking care of you can't always judge the difference between ordinary postoperative discomfort and a serious complication.

Err on the safe side and spend at least one and preferably two nights—with a private nurse—in a hospital or after-care facility. Even if the nurse doesn't perform any life-saving maneuvers, having one with you will calm your anxiety. "Now that I've been through it," said one woman I talked into staying overnight with professional nursing care (rather than going home under a friend's watchful eye), "I can't imagine how I could have gone home the same day."

Temperature and blood pressure need to be checked regularly. Vomiting is unpleasant and more than that, it's bad for your face. If you have nausea, your nurse can administer a fast-acting shot to control it. Cold compresses need to be applied constantly the first two days. It's trendy to use bags of frozen peas, but at the risk of being accused of being old-fashioned, spare me the lumpiness and the plastic wrapper. I like the feeling of tried-and-true gauze compresses dipped in ice water. And while the nurse is applying compresses and greasing the peeled or resurfaced skin, she can be vigilant for the unusual swelling and hardness that are signs of bleeding under the skin.

During my first few postoperative hours this time, I couldn't imagine walking the three steps to the bathroom. But by the middle of the night, I make the trip with help. I don't recognize myself in the mirror. Even though I've been through this before and am prepared for it, it's a shock. "Surprise and distress" is a common reaction, says Donna Phillips, a private-duty nurse who specializes in post–plastic surgery cases. Patients "seem to have skipped over this part, psychologically, in the pre-operative stage, perhaps in order to protect themselves from additional anxiety and fear." What's my excuse? I knew what I was getting into and I'm still horrified. Shiny brow. Blown-up eyelids and cheeks. Diaper on the tip of my nose. An upper lip the color of a blood orange. Slits for eyes. Because of the brow and nose and sinus work, I look even worse than I did after face-lift number one, if that's possible. In Phillips's experience, "Many patients say, 'If I'd known I would look like this, I never would have done it.' Luckily," she adds, "it's a transitory stage."

Completing the fashionable crash-dummy look is the gauze-helmet dressing. In theory, it keeps swelling down and protects the incisions around the ears. I know of a few doctors who don't believe in the helmet. And some claustrophobic patients can't tolerate it.

One group of face-lift patients who will never be without their mummy-wraps are characters in films. The headdress is a favorite image in the nearly 100 plastic surgery-themed films, including *Ash Wednesday*, the 1973 Elizabeth Taylor vehicle about a wealthy wife who undergoes a face-lift and other cosmetic surgery procedures to save her marriage. The film uses actual operation footage and lists a medical adviser in the closing credits, but there's nothing correct today about Taylor's character wearing her chapeau of bandages for *six weeks*. In real life, the helmet comes off the day after surgery or by the second day at the latest. As do the drains.

Two Jackson-Pratt drains with bulbous ends dangle from tiny incisions in the back of the head; the oozing blood and serum collects in the bulbs, which are emptied at eight-hour intervals. "We call them pocket-books," says Peggy Broderick, the Nurse/Manager of Plastic Surgery Patient Care Services at Manhattan Eye, Ear & Throat Hospital. "They're a shock to some people, but they're important because they ease the body's work so the fluid does not have to be reabsorbed."

The Gory Details

A lot of what I know about recovery, beyond my own personal experience and that of friends, I learned from Broderick. With her common-sense advice delivered in a soothing Irish brogue, she's better than Valium for a panicky patient. I first met Broderick after my first face-lift, when she came to my room, the second morning after my face-lift, to remove my blepharoplasty stitches. I lay in my bed, obsessing about how anyone could get the stitches out. I knew from my doctor's information packet that he would not be removing any stitches himself. "But don't worry," I was assured, "there is a woman here who does nothing but take out stitches. She takes them out for every surgeon on staff. She's better at it than the doctors." That woman turned out to be Broderick.

Broderick carries a special tool kit while making her rounds from patient to patient. Gauze sponges. Q-tips. Suture-removal kit (this includes scissors and disposable tweezers, an ophthalmology loop). And for recalcitrant stitches, a jeweler's forceps. After surgery, the cheeks are numb but the eyelids aren't. "They are very sensitive," says Broderick. "That's why I go carefully. I never had a stitch that didn't come out. The eyelid incisions heal so well. The eyelids are so forgiving." But, she warns patients, "your eyes won't close normally for a week."

She sat on the edge of my bed and told me not to be afraid. Then she put a pillow on her lap and my head on the pillow (a trick she learned from a predecessor who had a bad back and couldn't bend over). She warned me there could be pain, but there wasn't any. I closed my eyes and relaxed and in a matter of minutes, with the barest stings and the slightest tugs, the stitches were out. "Is that all there is to it?" I asked. "Why did I worry so much?"

It hurts loved ones more than it hurts the patient, says Broderick. "Boyfriends and husbands are like babies," she says. "They cannot watch when I take stitches out. They hate to see their women swollen and bruised and suffering." And the women? "They play the sympathy card to the hilt."

Pain may be the easiest postoperative symptom to deal with, thanks to modern day analgesics and sedatives. It's the other consequences—the swelling, the bruising, the sleep disturbances, the initial numbness and the subsequent tingling when nerves re-knit—that can be the most surprising, and for some, unsettling. "For several months after surgery one feels the nerves . . . waking up again, tickling or itching or buzzing a little," wrote *Designing Women* star Dixie Carter in her autobiography. "There is a feeling of tightness for a few weeks that goes away with the last bit of swelling, helped by the natural movements of your face."

Broderick says that when she tells patients that the discomfort is all normal and to be expected, "They'll say, 'But nobody told me.' " They need a lot of reassurance that the numbness in the face will disappear gradually. Even when they've been warned that numbness in the cheek and under the chin can last, though at a greatly diminished level, for up to six months or a year, many women are surprised when it doesn't go away sooner. In my own personal experience, the numbness didn't bother me— especially considering what it replaced—the jowls. Deep plane face-lifts and endoscopic brow lifts require the most patience. Broderick tells the endoscopic brow-lift patient, "Don't be surprised if you get swollen around the upper lids . . . you'll look like you had a terrible accident. You can say you ran into a plastic surgeon." Sounds like what happened to me.

Oddly, women who can spot a nose job across the room and who are veritable 411 operators regarding who did what to whom, may underestimate the recovery time needed following a lift. They see the experience in photographic terms as "before" (wrinkled and haggard) and "after" (refreshed and rejuvenated). They imagine their recovery as a two-week vacation to be spent at home cleaning closets, catching up on correspondence. It may well be. (But they'd better not be bending down and vacuuming, or working out with or without weights.) Why should they expect otherwise? After all, they've probably never heard anything different. Until recently, if patients had pain, swelling, temporary asymmetry, anxious moments, bad dreams, complications—they just didn't discuss it.

"Even the best-adjusted people go a little berserk when they see their swollen faces," says Broderick. They may feel they look like a freak. The body's two sides don't behave "the same way." One eyelid may droop more than the other. At this stage, she says, a wave of vulnerability may sweep over the patient. "They're afraid to touch their hair or their face." Part of Broderick's job is relieving their fears. "I tell them, 'You won't fall apart. Just avoid moving the neck muscles too much. Eat soft food. Avoid chewing.' I quietly assure them they'll be all right. I say, 'Nature takes over and does the recuperation for you if you just trust it. For heaven's sake, relax and you'll get better.' We would have no clientele if nature didn't do its business." Nonetheless, she says, some patients are "so panic-stricken, I have no voice left, calming them down."

She has learned that each patient's postoperative reaction is different. "One patient will say, 'It was easy as pie,' while another insists, 'I'll never do it again.' " And apparently breezing through your first face-lift—as I did—doesn't guarantee you'll breeze through the second one as easily. I didn't. And vice versa.

Sleeping on your back, in an elevated position—a further bleeding-control tactic and protection for the front-of-ear incision—is another annoyance. For some women, that's the hardest part of the experience. Some patients take the rules very seriously and sleep sitting up. "I think that's a cruelty," says Broderick. "Two pillows is enough. They're relieved when I say they don't have to lie on a pile of pillows for a week."

If Something Goes Wrong

Wednesday. Postoperative Day 1

On the first morning after surgery, I can sit up for a breakfast of oatmeal, although it's one of the few times I'll be awake today. I feel like Humpty-Dumpty, all head. My family has the privilege of walking me up and down the hall. I know I'm a sight because visitors who pass in the hall avert their eyes. Near the end of her shift, my private-duty nurse gets an emergency call—her child has burst an eardrum. I haven't lost my sense of priorities and, through my veil of sedation, I encourage her to leave. She arranges for another nurse to check on me. My appetite is back. Chewing is out of the question, but that's all right. Yogurt, applesauce, Jell-O, and mashed potatoes are comforting—vaguely reminiscent of when I was a kid and got out of going to school when I had a fever. The goal is to keep calm, so blood pressure won't go up. This is the most dangerous postoperative condition, since it can cause freshly cauterized blood vessels to bleed.

I was ignorant of such possibilities after my first lift. The academic bible on complications is *The Unfavorable Result of Plastic Surgery*. Ninety-five percent of the time, says its editor, Robert M. Goldwyn, nothing goes seriously wrong. Complications from facial procedures are statistically low and mostly reversible.

The most serious complications are bleeding, infection, and nerve damage. Though these occur rarely, and are usually correctable, they are still distressing. I'll explain why shortly.

Face-lift connected deaths "are few and far between, but they do occur," says Goldwyn. I'm well aware of that. I've reported on a few cosmetic surgery deaths.

A lot of people, myself included, had second thoughts about plastic surgery when they heard about what happened to the wife of singer James Brown. Adrienne Brown died in January 1996 after a lengthy operation that included several procedures including a face-lift and liposuction in an office-surgery facility. "How can cosmetic surgery leave someone dead?" asked Buddy Dallas, Mr. Brown's attorney. Good question.

The L.A. County Coroner's report concluded that Brown "had consumed [the illegal drug] PCP and several therapeutic medications while she had a bad heart and was weak from liposuction." That's one good reason for not taking your own drugs after surgery, but that's only one precaution.

In his Boston practice, says Goldwyn, "I warn every patient about death. But they don't think it applies to them. It feels very remote, just as when people get married, they don't believe they'll ever get divorced."

Why would anyone risk her life for a straighter nose or smaller hips? "There are a lot of things we do in the hope that it will make life better," says Goldwyn. "We all go on planes. Travel in Third World countries. Ride in cars. And we undertake elective surgery. All have small probabilities [of danger]. If someone has a tremendous fear, they don't go through with it."

There are probably one million cosmetic surgery procedures performed each year but there is no central data base of complications and deaths. In general, says Goldwyn, postoperative problems are often the result of a sequence of factors (judgments as well as techniques) that doom the enterprise to failure. All risks are increased when doctors perform multiple procedures, when a new procedure with a steep learning curve is performed by an inexperienced doctor, and when patients have preexisting health problems or withhold relevant medical data.

Lying about your age, for example, may seem a rather small transgression, but it can be a significant one. Doctors have found that patients who falsify their age are often the same ones who "forget" to mention their high blood pressure, alcoholism, drug abuse, diabetes, asthma, past heart attacks, and who may disregard pre- and postoperative instructions. They have stashes of their own pills, alcohol, and controlled substances. When nurses and recovery-house employees let their hair down, they tell hair-raising tales of patients who must be cajoled into surrendering their sleeping pills, booze, and cocaine. (It is illegal in many states to search a patient's belongings.)

Semantics are important when talking about unfavorable results. As patients, we label any unwanted or unexpected occurrence as a complication. Doctors sort them into neat categories:

Expected consequences are things one can count on, like incision scars, for instance, and the initial numbness and swelling.

Inevitable recurrences include the eventual return of sagging skin after a face-lift.

Disappointing anatomic results may be the specialty's biggest problem: a hated nose, an overly tight look.

While surgery that falls into these three categories may be disturbing, it is the *medical complications*, especially bleeding, infection and nerve damage, that are the most serious.

When real complications occur, patients tend to say, "Nobody told me." Often, however, they have been told but have forgotten. As Elizabeth Taylor said of all the possible complications described to her during the informed-consent ritual that preceded her recent brain surgery, "I know they're legally obligated to tell me, but I just don't want to hear these things. I want to bury my head under the blanket."

A study of twenty face-lift patients, ages forty to seventy, by psychologist Marcia K. Goin found that "however clearly the surgeon transmits the information [about complications], preoperatively," the patients—whether from denial, repression, fear or need for control—simply don't hear it. The patients' reactions ran the gamut from "It won't happen to me," to "I put them out of my mind"; "Nothing will happen to me because: 'I heal well'; 'I'm taking vitamin C'; 'I picked the right doctor'; or 'I'm afraid thinking about it will make it worse.' "

Patients, said Goin, had a near-magical faith in their own invincibility. "They tended to believe that while others might bleed excessively, they could somehow control their own bleeding."

Goin concluded that the patients simply didn't want to be deterred from having surgery. If they "truly believed that there was a real possibility that they might develop a facial paralysis as a result of an elective procedure, they could hardly allow themselves the indulgence" of surgery, she wrote. "So they refused to believe."

Beware of Your Medicine Cabinet

Bleeding after a face-lift is doubly annoying because it causes pain and delays the result of surgery. During the face-lift, dozens of tiny blood vessels are cut and sealed with electro-cautery. Occasionally—due to spikes in blood pressure—one capillary will burst its seal, causing blood to pool under the skin. That's called a hematoma. On average, 4 percent of face-lift patients develop one (men more than women, presumably because men have a stronger blood supply to the face due to their beards. Several years ago, when two prominent New York plastic surgery partners—both men—performed face-lifts on each other, it's said, they both got hematomas.) As we'll learn, the best treatment for this is prevention, though "There is no way you can prevent [hematomas] one hundred percent," says Boston plastic surgeon Eugene H. Courtiss, another authority on complications. Most hematomas occur within twelve hours of surgery, but they can occur up to two weeks afterward. The symptoms are severe, localized pain or hard and swollen tissue in the cheeks or in front of the ear, and a bluish discoloration.

After a face-lift, plastic surgery nurses check for hematomas by feeling inside the bandage helmet to determine if the skin is soft. "We use a finger test to see if we can get a finger under it," says Broderick. When patients ask her, " 'Suppose I get a hematoma,' " Broderick answers, " 'Did you ever stub your toe? It's blood trapped under the skin. Contact your surgeon and he'll release it. It's a minor inconvenience, not a disaster.' "

The blood can be removed with a syringe. In some cases, the doctor will take the patient back to the operating room and open the incisions (under anesthesia, of course). The resulting discoloration looks like a bad bruise and gradually disappears—but it can delay the return to normal by several weeks, making you look frightening all the while.

Hematomas can also be caused by vomiting (another reason why anti-nausea medication is given during and after surgery); by emotional upset; excitement; and exertion—or because the patient has a clotting problem or has been taking anti-coagulant medications, like aspirin. For all the patient's worry about the doctor's training, the anesthesia used, and the hazards of high technology, the patient can, in many ways, be her own biggest complication. Patients are cautioned to keep calm and avoid exercise, housework, and sexual activity—all of which can raise blood pressure. "I have to keep reminding patients to take it easy," says Broderick. "If they bend or have sex prematurely, they'll get more bruising. I tell them, 'Don't do anything to get heart pounding or racing. Your body is doing the work, don't intervene.'"

The recent play *Good As New*, a drama that uses a woman's face-lift as the catalyst for her confrontations with her husband and teen-age daughter, provided a graphic example of how *not* to behave after a face-lift. As the revelations and recriminations hit the fan, Mom, who had a face-lift that morning, becomes more and more agitated, bopping from lounge chair to bed. At one point she's crouched on the bed on all fours looking down at a photo album—a position that would be dangerous and painful to a real postoperative patient. If the jerky movements and lowered head didn't send the blood rushing to her face, the anger and upset would surely raise her blood pressure and cause postoperative bleeding. At least the mother doesn't ask for aspirin, a frequent culprit when there's bleeding.

No matter how many times pre-op patients are warned to avoid the seventy or eighty products containing aspirin (a blood thinner that interferes with clotting) for two weeks before (and after) surgery, many don't comply. When my friend "Colette" had a hematoma a few hours after her face-lift, a pain pill with blood-thinning effects was suspected. Colette, a New Yorker, chose a prominent surgeon in California. The operation went perfectly and Colette was spending the first night in her surgeon's recovery room, under a nurse's care. "I was asleep," recalls Colette, who has a history of hypertension. "My blood pressure must have spiked. A blood-vessel leaked on the side of my face. I opened my eyes in the middle of the night and saw one nurse showing the problem to another nurse."

Like most patients who suffer a complication, Colette wonders what caused it. Was it her thyroid condition? The estrogen she takes? Or the most likely suspect, two pain killers she took without permission? Warned not to take any aspirin products for two weeks before surgery, she had stopped her daily pills for chronic back pain. But two nights beforehand, she complained about her back to a friend who suggested Advil, which, though it contains no aspirin, has some aspirin-like effects. Without checking with her doctor, Colette took the pill twice before surgery. Whether it was the Advil or something else, there was bleeding. The doctor was called and early the next morning Colette was back in the operating room having the blood drained.

The residue was eventually absorbed, although, until it was, one side of her face was not a pretty sight. "There were days I thought I had gangrene as it turned every color and black," she says. "Other women would have been a pain in the ass, threatened to sue, cried, called their husband," says Colette, an exemplar of a maxim that patients are much more accepting of complications when their doctors are well-known. Instead, she applied compresses and kept calm. She was relieved no one had accompanied her out West. "That's all I needed," she says, "someone telling me, 'You shouldn't have done it.'" A few weeks later she was home in New York and the pain and discoloration were clearing up. In three months it was gone.

Colette's advice to anyone who gets a hematoma after a face-lift: "You should not worry. It only makes your blood pressure go up more. Remember, you picked that doctor because you had total confidence."

Delia is one patient who got a hematoma for no apparent reason. She followed instructions to a tee and, still, ten days after surgery, got a dreaded clot right in the middle of her cheek. Her doctor told her it could have come from coughing, sneezing or bending over. Even stress. "I have no explanation," says Delia, a Florida resident who had her surgery in Manhattan. "I developed this little problem on a Saturday." Thinking it was a bruise and not wanting to be a complainer, she applied ice and didn't contact the doctor until Monday. The blood was drained with a needle under local anesthesia. Later, a small section of her face-lift incision was opened, the bleeding was stopped and a tiny drainage catheter inserted.

Every day for four days, Delia returned for some more needle drainage. By the end of the week, she was told she was on her way to recovery and the dark bruise on her cheek would disappear in four to six week˙ (It did.) "I can live with that," says Delia. "It's a temporary inconvenience." 1 ˙e problem hasn't diminished her satisfaction with her face-lift.

The result may have been satisfactory, but waiting two days to call the doctor could be a disaster if there is bleeding after eyelid surgery. If you tear the blood vessels while removing fat, says Guy Massry, director of Oculo-Plastic Service, Annheiser-Busch Eye Institute, St. Louis University, "you get bleeding." Bleeders are cauterized during surgery. Very occasionally, the bleeding will start again. "Bending, stooping, and lifting after surgery increases blood pressure," says Massry. Bleeding in a closed space like the orbital cavity puts pressure on the optic nerve. The problem is evident, he says, "if the eyelid swells up like a baseball and becomes tense." This is a true medical emergency and the blood must be drained as soon as possible or the damage can be irreversible. It *can* cause loss of vision. The risk is four one-hundredths of one percent; there have been more than seventy-five such events in plastic surgery annals.

The most common complications of eye surgery are dry eye, incomplete closing of the eye, and a drooping lower eyelid. All can usually be treated or corrected.

If you've spent a year interviewing doctors and choosing just the right one, it's almost an affront to have a complication, but every surgeon in the world has them occasionally. The test of a doctor is how he or she handles them when they occur. Treatment should be aggressive and the doctor should be supportive. As Robert Goldwyn says, "The patient merits our sympathy. Someone who has had aesthetic surgery . . . frequently has sought it against the advice of family, friends, and other physicians and may have had to pay for it personally. When something goes wrong, he or she feels foolish, ashamed, guilty, and angry."

Infection after a face-lift is exceedingly rare because of the excellent blood supply in the face—but when it occurs, it is usually around the fifth day. When "Carla" came down with a virulent wound infection one day postoperative, she was terrified.

Carla seemed the last person who would be vulnerable to infection. But infections have their own logic. She was in excellent physical shape, fanatical about healthy eating and exercise, and so confident about her ability to snap back fast, she stayed only one night after surgery and refused to have a private nurse, even when the anesthesiologist told her before surgery, "There are times in life you should be a little extravagant." But that isn't Carla's nature.

The morning after surgery, after the helmet dressing and drains were removed, Carla was raring to go. She got her pills and instructions and was discharged. She took a cab home. No sooner had she walked in the door of her apartment, when she was suddenly overcome with uncontrollable vomiting. She dragged herself to the phone and called her doctor's office. The response she got probably saved Carla's life. The doctor was in the middle of the office hours and when the nurse took the call, she quickly relayed Carla's symptoms. He knew what had to be done. Carla wasn't told, "Take some Compazine and call me in the morning." The nurse said, "Don't move. I'm coming to get you and take you back to the hospital."

Carla couldn't have made it on her own. By the time she was back in her hospital bed, she had all the signs of infection—weakness, pain, swelling, and redness that was spreading down the side of her face and neck, her arm and torso. Her fever was 104. Cultures were taken, and intravenous fluids and antibiotics started. Treatment was aggressive. Her surgeon called in an infectious disease expert to identify the bacteria. It wasn't the staphylococcus strain that many people believe lurk in hospitals. It was a less common streptococcus infection.

Carla's surgeon said that in twenty years of practice, he had never seen an infection after a face-lift—he had only read about them in textbooks. No one knows what caused it. No one else on the operating schedule that day got an infection. By the fifth day after her operation, when the infection was getting worse, not better, Carla began to lose faith. "I really thought I was going to die. I felt very vulnerable. I thought the old man with the scythe was after me." But finally the massive infusion of antibiotics halted the spreading redness, and the infection began to retreat. Through it all, Carla's surgeon did not abandon her. He and several other physicians followed her every day. Carla spent thirteen days in the hospital with private nurses around the clock—at her doctor's expense. When she finally went home in a nurse's care, she still had blotchy redness in her cheek and neck, which subsided gradually, and a stiff neck—which was treated, again at her doctor's expense, by a physiotherapist. The aftermath was a temporary bout of thinning hair—a reaction of the hair follicles to all the antibiotics. Although she was able to return to work a month after surgery, she didn't feel like herself again for eight months. Only then could she enjoy the results of her face-lift. "The moral of the story," says Carla, "if you're going to have plastic surgery, do it in a hospital with a reliable doctor who is trustworthy and will take care of any eventuality—not someone who will try to hide the complication. Don't try to save money. Do the two-day stay. It's insurance." It's taken a while, says Carla, but "I've regained my confidence in the future and my safety."

The way patients respond to the stress of recovery has a great deal to do with their personality type, said the Goins. *Passive-dependant* types, who are normally compliant, may "regress to a clinging, smothering dependence" that may drive care-givers away. *Obsessive-compulsive* types "may invent complaints to compensate for feeling out of control." *Narcissistic* individuals, who place great importance on their physical appearance, may worry "constantly about minor swelling, bruising and discomfort," but once it has past, they can show an "exaggerated enthusiasm about the result." (Yikes, are they talking about me?) The *paranoid personality* may be the most difficult. "Belligerent and hostile patients sometimes have something very real to be belligerent and hostile about," say the Goins. But if the hostility is an "all-pervading" paranoid sort, it is likely to be made worse by surgery and will end unhappily for patient and surgeon. The paranoid patient may attack the hospital, unfairly, for its lack of "cleanliness . . . the nursing attendants for being rude and rough," and accuse the doctor of "turning over the operation to an assistant."

Keep Calm!

It's Thursday; two days after my surgery, and I'm supposed to go home this morning. My nurse does the honors on the helmet removal, snipping the bandages and gently removing the casing and then pulls out the vampire drains. Ouch. This is definitely a bad hair day. I look in the mirror and notice a roll of swelling on my right temple. Uh, oh. Dr. Z arrives and tells me the right side needed more lifting than the left. Rather than raise my hair line, he shirred the incision a bit on the temple. The swelling will shrink to fit, he says, and if it doesn't, there are remedies. I decide to worry about that tomorrow. Right now, my head feels like a large shiny coconut with two black eyes. Will I be able to hold it up for the short walk home? "You'll feel better when you're home," says the nurse. With her help, I slip into my jeans, cardigan, and loafers, and wrap a large scarf around my head, leaving a flap to hold in front of my face so only the eyes are exposed and they're covered with sun glasses resting loosely on my numb tender brow. I'm given my postoperative instructions—no bending, no exertion, no getting my nose dressing wet in the shower, sleep propped up, soft foods, call if you have bleeding or unusual pain—and told when to return to my doctor's office for stitch removal.

"Let's get out of here," says J, who can't bear hospitals. But before I am allowed to collapse in my own bed, I have to make it across the street to my sinus doctor's office to have the nose packing removed. Apparently I'm breathing through straws imbedded in the nasal packing, a great innovation since my previous sinus surgeries, when I had to breathe through my mouth till the packing was removed. The waiting room is filled, as usual, but I am whisked into a treatment room, so as not to frighten the other patients. There are benefits to looking horrendous.

The only way to describe what happens next is to say that what feels like two red alligators and the contents of the London sewer are pulled out of my nose. Don't ask. No wonder my head felt so heavy.

The sinus doctor is pleased with his interior handiwork and compliments me on the exterior work which is plastered in position with white tape. "Your nose looks good," he says reassuringly. "Dr. Z did a good job." I am incredulous that I can breathe through my nose again after months of blockage. "But who do I blame for all this swelling?" I ask. Naturally, he blames Dr. Z.

Home at last, our doorman, Raf, gives me a knowing wink. Manhattan doormen have seen it all. In my own bed, propped up on a stack of pillows, eating Jell-O, I feel much better—until my brother drops by and exclaims, "Oh my God. What a sight."

This is, of course, one reason why people go out of town for this surgery. I call a friend to say I'm alive and confess that I had more than my sinuses "done." From the tone of her voice, I think she had figured that out already. I wish I could wash my hair.

I make it to the dinner table. I've heeded the advice given by a friend before my first face-lift and stocked the refrigerator, in advance, with soft, low-sodium food (salt increases swelling, the friend had warned). I can hardly look at me. I'm more swollen than the last time, but there is less pain and bruising. I keep a chart to remind me when to take the various medications—antibiotic, anti-swelling, pain.

I warn everyone not to do anything that might promote stress. "Don't raise my blood pressure," I tell them before adding my favorite new medical word: "I don't want a hematoma." Having been through this before, I have most of the necessities on hand. But it says something about the increased popularity of face-lifting that Meridyth Webber, a housewife in New Jersey, has been able to make a business out of supplying post-face-lift kits to plastic surgeons. Webber includes a special contour pillow to keep the neck in the proper position; a grasping tool so you don't have to bend to pick up your socks; relaxation tapes (definitely not for me), a bell to summon help (to be used cautiously—not all husbands appreciate being rung for); a page-magnifier for those post-bleph blurry eyes; and a baby toothbrush and baby spoon. I have a few of the things on her list including flexible straws, hand mirror (the better to see myself), and small spoon for the temporary lockjaw. A day or two after surgery, such a kit could be more appreciated than a fruit basket.

The face-lift is a great equalizer. It's no cushier for a Pamela Harriman, our late ambassador to France, than someone less powerful. Harriman had the same postoperative experience as anyone else. According to Sally Bedell Smith's biography, "Pamela spent the night in the hospital, tended by a private nurse who applied constant ice compresses to reduce swelling, before moving to the apartment of her friend Kitty Carlisle Hart." Then, Harriman flew to her estate in Virginia for two weeks of recuperation. "Between the stitches and the inevitable swelling and bruising, her face looked monstrous at first." Harriman "stayed in bed, keeping her head elevated at all times, sleeping propped up on several pillows." Pain wasn't a problem for her. "Face-lifts are not usually characterized by postoperative pain. Instead, there is often a disconcerting numbness, and a sensation," according to one of Smith's sources, of "having a rubber band around your face. Your scalp feels tight and your jaw feels tight." Sounds right to me.

By *Friday* I can finally wash my hair, although it's awkward trying to keep the nose splint from getting wet. I put a shower cap over my face. I'd prefer to stay closeted, but life goes on. My presence is required in the lobby for a building committee meeting. I swath my head in a large scarf. Only my sunglasses are visible. Having forewarned my fellow members, they're solicitious. I receive pitying pats on the shoulder. Actually, the pain is minimal, thanks to the medication. But my ears ache from time to time, a typical complaint. Ever since my first lift, my ears have been slightly more sensitive to cold. Meridyth Webber ought to add earmuffs to her kit.

Sleep is fitful the first few nights if you're not used to sleeping on your back propped up. On the fourth night I wake up from a dream that I was ostracized at a picnic. Someone told me I was ugly, and that's exactly how I feel. J is solicitous but I notice he can't bear to look at me. My under-eyes are black and blue. I can read, but am having trouble concentrating. Despite daily shampooing, there's still some blood and gunk matted in my hair. My face is beginning to turn yellow. The upper lip is now brown and gritty. My lips are chapped and peeling. I notice a strange fold under the chin that worries me unduly. My face looks wider when it's supposed to be higher. When I attempt to raise my brow I feel something move on top of my head. Oh, my God, how far did he raise my forehead? My speech is slower. Some numbness in my lip makes it difficult to form words. I try to keep calm. You'd think I hadn't done this before. A friend who had a face-lift a month before calls to say she is rubbing her scars with Vitamin E. I wasn't given Vitamin E, but she has a scar across her scalp and I don't.

After dinner, Dr. Z calls. "I know about now you are feeling your worst," he says. I am overcome with gratitude. The man who put me in this state has some compassion. He is not abandoning me. He is the one person I feel I can complain to. I tell him I'm fine physically, but mentally a mess. What is this line under my chin? He says it sounds like swelling along a muscle. The neck was perfect when he closed me up; if it doesn't go away, it's easy to fix later. "Whatever is necessary will be done. Don't worry, you will look great," he assures me. I want to believe him.

But as I learned later, he's wrong about one thing. Although this is a bad day, it's not the worst. That is yet to come.

The Face-lift Blues

Many face-lift patients find themselves emotionally vulnerable during recovery. "All surgical procedures, even aesthetic procedures that the patient badly wants, are a source of emotional stress," wrote the Goins. In their study of postoperative anxiety, they wrote, patients "are placed in a situation in which they must depend on the surgeon, whom they may or may not trust. This . . . can activate old anxieties . . . or intensify existing intrapsychic conflicts." Coping mechanisms that "are adequate for most ordinary situations, can be disrupted, causing them to operate in an exaggerated or destructive fashion."

It's nice to know I'm not alone. What I'm feeling is fairly typical.

By Saturday, I give J the day off. My son is coming to keep me company. If my face scares him, he doesn't let on. My head feels sensitive around the stitches. When I press my forehead, I feel pain. I can't wait to have the stitches and the nose splint removed. I remember, after my first lift, finding the staples in the back of my head the biggest annoyance and counting the days till they were removed. They don't bother me as much this time. Although, it's shocking to realize that someone took a staple gun to your head.

"People are so frightened of staples—they don't want metal things in the head," says Peggy Broderick. "But I tell them they are the best for wound healing. Stitches in the hair are a nuisance. You get pulled hair. Staples don't damage hair follicles. They are so quick and easy to put in and take out."

I have other things to worry about. I have donuts of swelling around my eyes and a web of skin that stretches from my nose under my lower lid forming a little gutter below the inner corner of each eye. There are no visible cheek bones. I feel like a gourd. I'm sure there will be a hollow sound if I'm tapped. On the plus side, the hated horizontal lines on the bridge of my nose are gone along with the glabella crease (although a vestige of the vertical line is still there—like a wrinkle that won't press out. It can be peeled at a later date. Interestingly, I have minimal stiffness in my neck—much less trouble turning my head from side to side than after my first lift and less numbness under the chin. Every once in a while, crackles of nerve endings in my cheek sputter like lightning on the plains of Kansas. That's the nerves reconnecting. The swelling at my temple worries me.

Day 6. Today I'm supposed to wet the nose splint in the shower—in preparation for its removal. This is the moment of truth. J insists on escorting me to the doctor's office. I hope we don't bump into any acquaintances in the neighborhood. Dr. Z has a separate entrance for postoperative patients, but, still, I feel that bringing a husband into this fairly feminine waiting room is like bringing a man to a lingerie department. J stays in the anteroom while I am led to a treatment room. The nurse removes all but a few stitches at the base of my earlobe. Snip, snip. Tug, tug. I barely feel it. I point out the lumps of swelling that trouble me. "It's too soon to worry," she says. "The swelling is still there and it is often uneven." I had read in *Vogue* that it's painful when the nose tape is removed. I braced myself. But thanks to the pre-soaking and some miracle cement thinner applied by the nurse, the tape lifts off painlessly. Voilà. She hands me a mirror. A nice straight nose. It's a fraction of an inch shorter and not hanging over like a witch. But I don't recognize it as mine. And I certainly don't recognize the face.

"It's a great nose," she says.

"I'll have to get used to it," I answer. Was I expecting a magical transformation?

The nurse warns it will take three weeks to look okay and for the swelling in the nose to go down. But it will take a year for the internal nose swelling to subside and the final result to be visible. I know that one in five nose jobs require re-operation, but most doctors insist on waiting a year to do it.

I still have staples in my hair and dissolvable stitches dangling from my earlobe that give me a certain je-ne-sais-quoi quality. Nonetheless I'm making progress. I'm warned not to let my glasses rest on the bridge of the trimmer nose that now belongs to me. Tape them to your forehead, I'm told, but this proves to be awkward because the tape doesn't hold.

J doesn't flinch when I emerge from the treatment room, but he is noncommittal. He says he's waiting for the total package before commenting. I'm still not allowed to wear makeup or go to the hairdresser for two more days, when the staples come out. What's my hurry? It's not even one week. But a friend is being honored in a few days and I'm anxious to attend the dinner. J warns that I am putting undue pressure on myself to look presentable. "Send regrets," he says. But I don't want to.

Back home, I show my new nose to my mother, who happens to live next door. I know she'll tell me the truth. She's surprised. She likes it. "But your ears are big," she says. "It's a sign of intelligence."

I think they're just swollen.

Today, for the first time, I don't need a pain pill during the day. Only at night. My stepson visits. "Wow, you're going to be great." I suspect he's being diplomatic. I'm turning yellow and blue now, less red. Later I study my face at length in a hand mirror, trying to get familiar with it. Donna Phillips is right when she says, "All the reassurance and encouragement of friends and family won't give patients hope until the mirror begins to." Frankly, if this weren't so-called research, I would feel horribly guilty for all this self-involvement.

After a full week, the family is beginning to banter nervously about my nose. "It's turned up too much," says the step-daughter who was against the operation in the first place.

"Don't worry. It's still swollen. Soon it will look like Joan Rivers's nose," I joke. A friend calls and asks, with a slight edge in her voice, "Well, can you breathe?" Her insinuation: I didn't really need a nasal operation.

Feeling is starting to return to my face. My cheeks and forehead are tender and numb. I have a story due about an L.A. plastic surgeon and have scheduled a phone interview with him. I realize during the conversation that my speech is a little slower because my upper lip is not working as well as it should. By way of apology, I mention my "condition." He kindly warns me to expect a depression now. Expect it? I've already got it. Along with trouble breathing, achy ears, achy forehead, swollen face, blue circles under the eyes. Now that the splint is off, the nose is growing. The upper lip is red and raw. I have no smile lines, which makes me look like a doll. I know from experience they'll come back. I also know from experience, that the swelling will go down, but somehow, when you're in the middle of the healing, you find it hard to believe that's where you're headed.

On *Day 8*, I am to discover that the sinuses get worse before they get really better. Breathing today is impossible. My peeled upper lip is still red. This morning I'm due to have the last staples removed from the back of my head. I insist on going to the doctor's office alone. I'm not an invalid. I wear my usual disguise. But I'm not feeling perky. I'm a woman on the edge of a nervous breakdown. In the lobby, as I head for the door, a woman engaged in conversation with the doorman stops in mid-sentence to gawk at me. "Would you please stop staring at me," I snap. The doorman inquires if I'm feeling any better. "No!" I say emphatically.

I'm carrying a new item of camouflage: a pleated paper fan to hide my greased red lip. But it just calls more attention to my condition. By the time I arrive at Dr. Z's office I'm on the verge of tears. What's my problem? I had my sinuses fixed and I can't breathe. I can't read without my glasses and I hate taping them on my forehead. My hair's a mess. I'm worried that my face is overdone, I can't decide whether I like my nose or hate it. And I feel very guilty about complaining. It's like bitching about having indigestion after a meal at a four-star restaurant. You're lucky to even be going to dinner there. Why did you eat so much?

The staple removal is a non-event. When the fifteen or twenty annoying metal staples used to close the incisions in the hair in the back of the head are popped out, there are only twinges of pain and great relief. The nurses who do this postoperative aesthetic work are professionals.

The stitches closing the five, one-inch brow-lift incisions in the top of my head will absorb. But those stitches are not the ones that hold the brow—or "fixate" it, in medical jargon—in its new higher position. Several techniques are used for fixation, and surgeons spend a great deal of time debating whose technique is best.

My brow was raised (like a window shade that pulls up from the bottom) with a hoisting system of hidden guy lines tunneled under the scalp that will eventually be absorbed. The surgeon pulls the cords and the brow is raised to the right height, then secured in place. But some physicians yank up the brow manually, temporarily anchoring it in position with tiny titanium screws. The screws are removed a few days later with a special screwdriver. Some women freak out at the thought of having screws in their head. But whether it is staples, stitches, or screws—for a month or two after a brow-lift, you may feel like a ventriloquist's wooden-headed dummy.

Once the stitches and staples and screws are out, you're ready for a beauty treatment. My surgeon has an aesthetician on staff and I'm offered complimentary makeup. The surgeon benefits as much from this service as the patient does, since bruised-looking patients don't help any doctor's reputation. What I really need today is therapy. As it turns out I get some, along with the makeup, when I settle into the aesthetician's reclining chair. She assures me I'm not a gargoyle. "You look amazing for the eighth day," she says. She's never seen anyone do so well so soon. Almost no bruising, only under the eyes, which, partisan that she is, she blames on the sinus surgery.

Armed with perhaps a bit too much concealer and eyeshadow, I decide to venture to the hairdresser and bump into a pal from L.A. exiting as I enter. She wouldn't have recognized me in my scarf, dark glasses, and donut-hole eyes, but I foolishly say, "Hi, Annie."

"Oh, my God," she says, focusing. "Didn't you just have this done a few years ago?" I must have had "neurotic recidivist" written all over me. At what point does one qualify as a scalpel slave?

Chastened, I quickly turn my back when I spy a former colleague. I am hustled into a private booth. A shampoo person with a gentle touch is summoned. Many doctors will send postoperative patients to a special salon for post-surgery shampoos, but I don't feel it's necessary. You just need a head washer with a light touch. A private cubicle helps too. My hair stylist is understanding. In half an hour I feel like a new person. I still look embalmed, but attractively. Patience is the only cure for that.

I feel confident enough to walk home and risk encountering friends. I invite my mother to have a look. "Oh my god," she says, "you're so pretty. So brave. So determined."

Still, I have to agree with J, I'm not ready for my closeup. I beg off attending a meeting at the office, saying "it could give plastic surgery a bad name," and send my regrets to the group honoring my friend. A trip to the sinus doctor reveals why I'm not breathing. This time it's the Venice sewer that has to be removed through my nose. But, I know I'm getting better. Today I can smell fragrance. The last time I had my sinuses repaired, it took three years to recognize perfume. During that sensory drought, I interviewed a cosmetic mogul who wanted my opinion of her latest scent. I apologized, explaining I had had sinus surgery and could not smell perfume. She confided that she had once had the same problem and her sense of smell had eventually returned. Miraculously, mine did, too.

Day 9. For the first time, I *feel* like working. I solve the eyeglass problem with new feather-light wire-framed eyeglasses that don't rest on the nose. Liberation. (It augers well that granny glasses no longer make me look like a granny.) Today my mother calls me "cute," and says, "I told your brother he will never recognize you." What does that mean? I realize I'm becoming extremely sensitive and paranoid. But it's not my lower face that bothers me. It is the tender nose and brow area.

On *Day 10,* J decides I need a weekend in the country. I remember, after my first lift, the anxiety of my first postoperative car ride. Suppose there's a short stop, I brooded. Would my stitches open up? No, they wouldn't. Just to be on the safe side, I took a pillow along and kept it in my lap. This time around, I don't feel so much like a china doll. I'm just impatient. My swelling is lopsided and my lip is puffed out like a blowfish. We stop at a fruit stand and the farmer takes one look at me and, instinctively, rubs his upper lip. Back at our weekend house, I lean over the kitchen counter to plug in an appliance and bang my forehead on the corner of the range hood. I panic. Everything was going so well, and now I'm sure I'm going to get a hematoma. I burst into tears. J warns me crying will just make me more swollen and fixes a makeshift ice pack.

I'm like a first-year medical student, imagining she has every condition in the textbook. Maybe the reason I was so much less nervous after my first face-lift was that I didn't have a clue, then, about what could go wrong, even though I'm sure I was warned.

That's quite typical. A study done at Vanderbilt Medical Center in Nashville examined how much information patients could remember after a detailed briefing about the risks (bleeding, infection) and possible postoperative results (pain, non-success) of the procedure they were about to undergo. Overall, the researchers found, there was only a 35 percent retention rate. Patients who considered themselves very nervous retained a bit more. Those who were calm retained less because they were more trusting.

Later, when I check my city answering machine, there's a soothing message from Dr. Z. "How are you doing?" Does he really want the truth? Rationally, I know I'm right on schedule and the swelling is expected. But emotionally, I'm sure I'll never look normal again. What did my mother mean when she called me cute? I don't want to look cute. I am not pining for my old nose, but it's obvious I haven't bonded with my new one yet.

This kind of postoperative nose anxiety can be a serious problem for plastic surgeons. According to San Francisco plastic surgeon Mark Gorney, the most dangerous patient is the single, adult male who is immature, narcissistic, and has a neurotic fixation on his nose. Four plastic surgeons have been murdered by men who had had nose surgery, and male rhinoplasty patients figure prominently in accounts of threats to plastic surgeons.

To screen patients who are prone to dissatisfaction or violence, Robert Goldwyn, the Harvard plastic-surgery professor, advises colleagues to be wary of the patient:

> who writes an excessively long letter to arrange the initial consultation;

who is rude or demanding or unkempt;

who makes the doctor's office her (or his) home;

who praises the doctor excessively and denigrates the doctor's
colleagues;

who gives a false history;

who schedules and reschedules an operation without good reason;
i.e., a cold or a death in the family;

who refuses to be photographed;

who wants an operation to please someone else;

who is paranoid or depressed;

whose spouse says no (adamantly); and

whom the doctor dislikes.

Sometimes doctors don't see the problem until it is too late. In 1991,
Dr. Selwyn Cohen, a plastic surgeon in Bellevue, Washington, a wealthy
suburb of Seattle, was shot to death in his office by Beryl Challis, sixty,
who said she was experiencing pain from a face- and especially a brow-
lift he'd performed a year before. After murdering Cohen, Challis killed
herself.

Day 11. The top of my head feels like wood. My lip is still red and puffy
and, now, the tip of my nose is sore. The friend (whose testimonial dinner
I missed) figures out the real cause of my doldrums. "The pain pills are
making you paranoid," she says. She's right, of course. Why didn't I think
of that?

The Turning Point

Day 12. After a night without narcotics, everything looks better. I wake
up optimistic. I decide to retire the pain killers for good. The swelling is
coming down. I study my nose in a three-way mirror and like it. But I
worry that J hates it and won't say so. "That's not true," says one step-
daughter, interpreting. "He just hasn't decided yet." Uh-oh.

Day 13. Dr. Z's office calls. The doctor wants to see me at the hospital. He must be reading my mind. Peggy Broderick assures me I look great for less than two weeks. Dr. Z says he is pleased with my progress. Nose still swollen—"it will drop a little." Face is swollen. He can feel where I dented my skull on the stove hood, but there was no bleeding. He prescribes hydrocortisone for my lip. Later, a neighbor tells me I look wonderful. Still slightly paranoid, I wonder, Is she humoring me?

Day 14. The magic two-week mark. If I had had just a face-lift, I could probably face the world without embarrassment. I'm going public this week, but I still don't feel ready for scrutiny. Without makeup, these bruises under my eyes (from the brow lift, from the rhinoplasty, from the sinus? Who knows) look like the black under-eye warpaint worn by football's New York Jets. Dr. Z's aesthetician has offered to do my makeup every day, but I like being independent. I slink over to Boyd's, the Madison Avenue beauty-product supermarket, and invest seventeen dollars in a pot of banana-colored cover-up cream. I imagine I look like a battered wife, but the saleswoman wasn't born yesterday. "How long ago did you have it?" she whispers. "Only two weeks? You look great." In appreciation, I purchase a few more items. I guess she earned her commission. I've cut way down on pain pills. Several pals want to see the results. Using a cooking metaphor, my stock answer is "I'm not done yet."

It is probably a smart decision. This is still a vulnerable time. If *my* experience is any barometer, about now, you may find yourself spending an inordinate amount of time with your mirror, in guilty vanity, studying your new face. As you feel more confident you will test the face, cautiously, on family and friends. This is a curious phenomenon. More than with any other cosmetic procedure, says Robert Goldwyn, "The opinions of others, even strangers, may greatly influence the patient's satisfaction." You swore you underwent this operation for yourself. You told the doctor you didn't want to look different, just fresher. But, now, you find yourself craving approval—and at the very least, hoping not to encounter disapproval. Steel yourself.

According to Goldwyn, a repository of wisdom on the subject,

" 'Friends' are diabolical assassins who delight in shooting verbal harpoons into [the] already surgically wounded patient." Frequently, says Goldwyn, one week after surgery—a highly vulnerable time—the patient will say to him, " 'Doctor, someone asked me why I have more swelling on one side than the other.' " Another scenario is the patient who complains that her friend looked " 'better in two days than I do, now, at two months.' " That may be true, but the women who took longer to recover may have had a more extensive operation that could last longer than the lift of the friend who recovered so quickly.

"Killer Karen" is Goldwyn's nickname for the friend who gasps and blurts out, " 'What did he do to you? He was supposed to be the best.' " While " 'Murderous Mary' " may ask, " 'When are you going to have your face-lift?' "

The girlfriend factor is hard enough to deal with when one has a lift and the other doesn't. Imagine how difficult it could be when they have the face-lifts at the same time. Often, I hear women encouraging friends to join them in surgery—for moral support. They say, "We'll share a room and recuperate together." It sounds like fun, but suppose one person has more swelling or develops bleeding or an infection. She feels like a failure. Her friend got the good face-lift and she got the complications. The buddy system is probably not a great idea.

Going Public

Day 15. The earlier a patient goes out in public, the thicker her skin must be. No wonder I'm tense. If you think Killer Karen and Murderous Mary are formidable, imagine facing 400 plastic surgeons at a scientific meeting at the Waldorf. I don't fool anyone in this crowd with my dark glasses. Their solicitousness is collegial, but it embarrasses me.

"You're going to look great," says one physician. "How are you feeling?" inquires another.

"How do you know?" I ask.

"I was working in the next operating room during your operation."

I find it disloyal to discuss my operation with anyone but my own doctor, so I don't share.

"Let's look at you," says another doctor acquaintance, taking my face in his hands. "Dr. Z did a good job," he says, in front of a group. I want to fall through the floor.

Day 16. I've been religiously following instructions and sleeping on several pillows, but somehow I wake up flat on my back with a big pain in the top of my head. So that's why they want you to sleep propped up—to keep the blood from pounding in the top of your head. The scabs are beginning to fall off the scars behind my ears. I still feel thatches of sticky hair where the staples were removed. I can raise my eyebrows today. This is good news and bad news. Does this mean my forehead is dropping already? I decide the lip peel coverup I bought is the wrong color. What was I thinking? I should have worked this out before surgery. At the Waldorf, I stop at every post-surgery makeup booth in the medical-exhibits area and pick up samples of coverup. Bio-Medic's is the best color and texture. It stays put—especially when you set it with powder—and provides good coverage without looking like latex. Salespeople at the booths, recognizing the post-surgical look, offer me an arsenal of post-peel soaps and lotions to try.

Several doctors, meaning well, can't resist offering advice, which I take as subtle criticism. One tells me I should come to his clinic and he'll laser my glabella crease. A South African surgeon warns that my hair will fall out in three months from the screws used in the endoscopic brow-lift (I didn't have screws). Another doctor has decided my smile is crooked and I have nerve damage. (I have some very anxious days before I can discuss it with Dr. Z.)

Nerve weakness from a face-lift, though infrequent and usually temporary (in one study of 6,500 lifts—there were fifty instances, only seven of them permanent), can be devastating.

Many women fear their nerves will be cut purposely. The worst-case scenario, says plastic surgeon Daniel Baker, is if the facial nerve—which lies under the SMAS in the cheekbone area—is severely damaged. Then one whole side of the face could be paralyzed. The risk of complications is greater in new face-lift techniques that involve deep tissue manipulation, especially when a doctor is less familiar with the technique. But most nerve injury comes from *bruised* nerves, not *severed* nerves and is temporary. An uneven smile caused by weakness on one side of the lower lip is almost always transitory and usually won't last long.

If there had been permanent injury, I could expect little sympathy. Everyone from bosom buddies to family members to jurors in malpractice suits are prone to say, "You asked for it." Passing along a cautionary tale of a woman who died of a tummy tuck, a mid-Western acquaintance says, "She died of vanity. No doctor here would touch her face and stomach because she was seventy. So some other woman got her diamond ring."

Most of the time everything goes well; 90 percent of patients are happy. "If a healthy person goes to a qualified, trained doctor and has a cosmetic operation in an approved facility, the degree of safety is very, very high," says Eugene Courtiss.

Day 20. In *Ash Wednesday,* Elizabeth Taylor's character says she's heard it takes three weeks to get used to your new face. That's the movies. From my experience, if a nose is involved, it takes a bit longer. Today my doorman says, "Looking good." J sees improvement, too, but says, "You're not there, yet." I'd like to stay in my stateroom till we get there. Happily, I have a deadline to meet, and for the first time since surgery I sit down at the computer and forget my face.

Day 21. Maybe Liz Taylor's character is right, after all. Today, even my critical stepdaughter is beginning to relent. "Well, finally, you have a chin. You were a grapefruit. You're getting there." The tentative approval works wonders. I dream I'm feeling better. I wake up feeling I've entered a new phase. Sleeping on my back isn't necessary anymore, but my cheeks are tender and I find a small, extra-soft goose-down pillow in the linen closet. I notice cotton pillowcases leave crease marks on my face, so I invest in a satin case. I like it so much I decide to give satin pillowcases to any friends having face-lifts.

Day 22. The stitches under my earlobes have dissolved. Finally, today, I'm allowed to color the five-week growth of roots. Why is no hair dying allowed? No wonder I've been depressed. The only tender spots on my face are close to my ears and the eyebrows.

Day 23. That was yesterday. Today, the top of my head is throbbing. I feel as if a brick had been dropped on it. Concerned, I call Dr. Z's office and am told to come right over. Several of the "befores" in the waiting room peek at me from behind their magazines. When my turn comes, I ask if I'll lose my hair and whether I have nerve damage.

Dr. Z calms my fears and, by raised eyebrow and a shake of the head, communicates his displeasure at his colleagues. "If you lose any hair, you'll be my first endoscopic-brow patient who did," he says. Regarding nerve damage, we look at my pre-op pictures and I make a broad smile for him. The lower lip drops a little lower on one side than the other. But I have no trouble puckering and grimacing. "You do not have nerve damage," he assures me. "A little temporary numbness on one side. It will go away soon." (It does in two weeks.) The pain in the top of the head is not unusual after the endoscopic brow-lift, he says. "Take Advil for a few days," he says.

Day 24. I'm suddenly interested in experimenting with makeup, as a way to disguise the remaining imbalances caused by swelling. A makeup artist friend gave me a list of suggestions and I take it to Bloomingdale's. All sales resistance has vanished. Nothing is too good for my face. At home with my purchases, I try everything and naturally end up with irritated eyes. This is dumb. Now I need a prescription for ophthalmic ointment.

Day 25. From now on, J has something good to say almost every day.

Day 26. My internist calls to inquire about my recovery. She has a medical interest and perhaps a personal one. I stop by her office for a once-over. She admires the result wholeheartedly, until she learns I'm taking Advil. "When you burn a hole in your stomach, I'm the one who is going to have to take care of you," she scolds. "Pain is good for the soul. And don't take Aleve, it causes palpitations." Back to plain Tylenol.

Day 27. The throbbing in the top of my head has subsided. (It's some comfort to learn, when interviewing New York plastic surgeon Paul Lorenc, that he tells his endoscopic brow-lift patients, "They'll feel as if they walked into a door.") Now I don't have any pain unless I press the top of my head. There's nothing left to obsess about except my lip. I am over-treating myself with all the samples of post-peel remedies and coverups. The lip should be healed by now, and instead it seems to be getting worse. A cortisone cream is prescribed. It works. The redness subsides.

One Month
I take the day off to attend a party to celebrate the ninety-ninth birthday of my aunt (did I mention that longevity runs in my family?). She tells me I look "beautiful," but, then, her vision isn't what it used to be. In the party pictures taken today, I look like just like Debbie Reynolds. That's fine if you're Debbie Reynolds. I'm not.

Four and a Half Weeks
"You're looking better today," says J, sounding markedly relieved. "When you smile, I can see what you're going to look like. I never lost hope, but, oh, what you do to yourself."

Five Weeks
J glances up from his paper at breakfast and says, "You look immeasurably better." On the way to a meeting, I bump into my mother who greets me with an approving kiss. She seems relieved too. "You're beautiful." At *Allure*, a colleague looks me over and tells me frankly, "You look like you've had something done." I appreciate her honesty. It's less unnerving

than noncommittal silence. When nothing is said, you feel like an actor in a flop.

A small comfort: my stepson reports someone saw me on the street and reported that I looked like a younger version of myself. My stepdaughter, meanwhile, is unrelenting about my nose.

When you're constantly being assessed, you are constantly assessing yourself. And now I have a new concern. I am certain I am developing a hairline scar on my upper lip. This seems beyond trivial after reading my friend Laura Landro's harrowing account of her survival from leukemia and a bone marrow transplant in The Wall Street Journal. But, then I tell myself, I'm trying to survive premature aging—which is a different kind of death sentence. Call me vain. Call me plastic. I am not ready to look like Miss Marple.

Six Weeks
A major breakthrough. This morning J announces he prefers the new nose to the old one. Vindication. Relief. But the lip scar is not getting better. If this infinitesimally small mark is driving me crazy, I can only imagine what a larger blemish would do to a person's self-confidence. I've learned that there is always a chance of scarring with any face peel—whether you've had dermabrasion, acid, or laser resurfacing. The good news is, scars are treatable. Off I go to Dr. Z. He agrees that a scar could be forming. I'm grateful he doesn't tell me it's my own fault—which it may well be, for trying all those different remedies. He gives me a shot of Kenalog, a steroid, in the lip. It has to be used sparingly or the tissue can wither. We discuss a new over-the-counter Vitamin E cream from Canada. He says he'll send for it.

On my way out, Peggy Broderick, who has probably seen more distraught postoperative face-lift patients than anyone in the country, puts these small concerns in perspective.

"I tell everyone you won't feel like yourself for six weeks and you won't *look* right for three months," she says.

"But," I respond, "the textbooks say a TCA peel should be healed in five to eight days."

"And I'm the Queen of England," she says.

Six Weeks Plus One Day

The tide has definitely turned. The face is falling into place. The askew smile is symmetrical now. "You're beginning to look good," says J. I no longer feel my brow is on top of my head. I can raise my eyebrows and express concern without knitting my brow. The nerves in the scalp are waking up. The incipient scar (which I must confess is no thicker than an eyelash) is subsiding. I still have residual numbness at the base of my nose. The left side of my head still feels wooden. But the right side feels normal now. My scalp is itching, which means the nerves are waking up. I'd be nervous if I didn't know it was to be expected.

Six Weeks Plus Two Days

Today I feel like I'm Miss America. We're on our way to a party and J turns to me as if he's seeing me for the first time and says, "You look really pretty." At the gathering, friends I haven't seen all year are complimentary. "You look different." "You look younger." "Did you change your hair?"

Nine Weeks

The lip is still red in three tiny spots, smaller than freckles, that are easily concealed with makeup. But I'm sure I'm developing a scar and stop in show it to a dermatologist. "What scar?" she says. She can't see it. The Vitamin E cream arrives from Canada. I'm told that, in some cases, it has gotten rid of twenty-five-year-old scars.

Three Months

Peggy Broderick predicted it to the day. Is it the Canadian Vitamin E cream or time? The lip is healed. No redness. No scar. No shiny scar tissue. The swelling in the temple is way down. (Subsequently, Dr. Z, using the tiniest cannula, got rid of the remaining swelling with liposuction, under local anesthesia in his office.) J doesn't pay attention to my face anymore. I've stopped obsessing. I study a picture of me on J's desk, taken when I was twenty (we've known each other since high-school). I don't recognize that girl, but I recognize her youthful nose. And, I'm happy to say, it's back on my face.

Some Time Later

The phone rings. It's a plaintive call from "Sunny" an old friend from another city, who deliberated for years about a face-lift. To do it or not to do it? This doctor or that doctor? I wondered if she would ever commit.

"I did it," she says. "And I know I've made a terrible mistake. I look horrible." She had the operation here in New York and is recuperating at a local hotel. Her surgeon has been attentive. He even came to the hotel to take out her stitches. I'm impressed.

"How many days has it been?" I ask.

"Five."

"Well, then," I say, like the veteran I am, "you're right on schedule. About now you should be feeling your worst."

A few months later, she sent a note saying she was fully recovered and happy with her results.

Nine

METAMORPHOSIS—
THE BUTTERFLY EMERGES

"Obviously, it's not a good thing to tell the truth."
—CHER.

Four months after the second face-lift, I have a dream—a nightmare, really. My face is back to the way it was—my old nose, my furrowed brow. When I wake up, I'm in a cold sweat. I rush to the mirror. Thank goodness, it *was* a dream. But what was I saying to myself in it? That I really wanted a more profound change and felt disappointed? That I'd hoped the face-lift would literally turn back the clock, rather than merely giving the appearance of having done so? I wouldn't be the first face-lift patient who expected real magic.

Whatever my subconscious is up to, one thing is clear: I don't want the old face back. But obviously, I haven't fully integrated the new look into my image of myself. That's the next phase and it may take weeks or even months. As the swelling goes down, the scars heal, the discoloration abates, and the stiffness in my neck eases, the familiarization process will take place—but all that will include hundreds of stolen glances in every mirror and reflective surface I pass.

Because the changes wrought by a face-lift are usually minimal and essentially recreate a previously existing condition, the new look should be easily integrated into one's self-image. Indeed, according to the Goins, the wrinkled and sagging facial and neck skin caused by gravity during aging "is never fully incorporated into the body image" of the patient, and therefore she shouldn't have a tremendous adjustment when the sagging skin is lifted and tucked out of the way.

As the wrinkles crept up on you and the cheeks slipped down over your jaw, you avoided looking at that face. That was a stranger's face, an image so incongruous with your picture of yourself, you refused to accept it.

Most face-lift patients have an idealized vision of themselves—and it's not necessarily at sweet sixteen. It's usually a more grownup face, maybe a picture of yourself from ten years ago. That's the face you hope to retrieve with the face-lift. That's the picture I carried around from doctor to doctor when I was shopping for my first face-lift. The face that followed that ideal moment was probably never incorporated into your body image, as I can attest. Since you never accepted that lax, lined face as your own, the theory is, the face-lift shouldn't require getting used to. But embracing one's rejuvenated self requires admitting that the former face needed fixing. And that's an admission not everyone can make.

Two months after her lift, "Lois," a political analyst, seems fixated on how attractive she was *before* the surgery. "I looked pretty good for fifty-seven," she tells me. Lois is one of those enviable people who always look well-tended despite traditional responsibilities of home-family-social life and a demanding career. More recently, she prided herself on aging better than most of her friends. The only thing she didn't like about herself were the deep smile lines. If she hadn't been allergic to collagen, she says, she could have had injections of it to plump up the troublesome lines and wouldn't have needed a face-lift at all.

Now that Lois has had the lift, the compliments she has been receiving are colliding with her carefully nurtured illusion that she really didn't need surgery at all, although no one—certainly not her husband—talked her into having it. It was her own decision and, like many women who opt for a face-lift, she timed it to an important event: her daughter's wedding. So now Lois feels defensive about her former face. Rather than accept the compliments, she focuses on the annoyances of recovery—the temporary complication she suffered that made her vision blurry for several weeks and undermined her feeling of competence.

"This has not been a happy experience," she says, downplaying what certainly appears to be a successful aesthetic outcome. It's as if by admitting improvement, she is devaluing her former self. Carefully choosing the most underwhelming tribute, she says, the result of the face-lift "is nice, but my head feels like it's in a vise. I have pressure on the temples. In the beginning, I felt like I had tape under my chin. My neck felt tight. Did I love that? No. I couldn't drive. All these nerve endings were crying for attention. Then, I'd see myself in the mirror and I looked great. My husband was supportive. He kept reinforcing how good I looked. He said, 'Your neck really looks great.' "

Lois pauses, before adding peevishly, "I hadn't ever noticed my neck *wasn't* great."

The simple fact is that accepting the new you requires admitting you were dissatisfied with the preoperative you. "Serena," a much photographed former jet-setter in her sixties, is quite willing to admit that before her recent face-lift she wasn't so alluring. "I found my 'before' pictures. I was flabbergasted. The difference is night and day. I feel rejuvenated. It's like having a second chance in life, looking the way you like to look again but still having the maturity. Now I look the way I feel," she says. "I feel I'm unbeatable, as if I could achieve whatever I wanted. As superficial as a face-lift sounds, it has made it possible for me to think young again."

Better Than Prozac?

After hearing all the pros and cons, and from the happy campers as well as the people with lingering complaints or unexpected complications, you have every right to ask, as many people do: How many people are happy or unhappy with the results of a face-lift?

A woman who frames this question in a negative way, I suspect, is hoping this is one expensive item of consumption she doesn't need. She'd like to cross it off her list with a pithy, "Been there. Considered that. Skipped it. Too many unhappy people."

Milton T. Edgerton's three-decade study at Johns Hopkins University of body dismorphic disorder—the individual who, in Edgerton's words, "feels trapped in the wrong face and wants a completely different appearance"—furthered the impression that the cosmetic surgery

patients are bizarre. Long before Michael Jackson's many nose operations, Edgerton was dealing with extreme requests—for instance, the
man who wanted to look like Johnny Carson. Such patients were routinely turned away by plastic surgeons. "We decided as long as we could
safely do what they asked, we would do it—even of it seemed excessive,"
says Edgerton.

It took fifteen different operations over a twenty-year period for the
Johnny Carson wannabe to achieve satisfaction with his appearance. "He
looks a little like Carson," says Edgerton, but, as the study proved, "it's
not how we look to others, it's how we *think* we look to others. After a
while," said the doctor, "we learn to stop making value judgments. A tiny
change can be a dramatic life-enhancing experience, while [what the
physician believes is] a miraculous improvement can mean little or
nothing to another person." In a series of several hundred cases, 25 percent of them male, "the vast majority were rehabilitated so they could
enjoy life." The bottom line in aesthetic surgery, says Edgerton, is no matter what others think of the changes, the patient is the only one who can
judge the success of his makeover.

It's only recently that the desire for cosmetic surgery has been considered as normal, not an indication of maladjustment. A study of postoperative attitudes, undertaken at the Robert Wood Johnson Medical School in
New Brunswick, New Jersey, found that cosmetic surgery makes people
happier. It "has a measurable positive, psychological effect," said plastic
surgeon Gregory Borah. Patients reported "less depressive symptoms,
improved quality of life outcomes, enhanced body image, improved well-
being." Predicts David B. Sarwer, a psychologist at the University of
Pennsylvania's Center for Human Appearance, "We're moving away from
considering it as 'trivial vanity,' and beginning to see it can be adaptive,
life-enhancing. As more baby boomers consider face-lifts, you'll see it
more accepted."

The motivations for restorative procedures such as the face-lift or eye-
lift vary from person to person. These patients generally like their appearance and want to maintain it, says Sarwer. What's more, he found, the
majority of face-lift patients are normal, psychologically—"no more neurotic than those who care about their haircuts"—and quite pragmatic

about the benefits of looking good. "We live in a society, where, like it or not," says Sarwer, "appearance matters in every social situation—the nursery, the courtroom, job interviews, partner selection. Those perceived as more physically attractive reap benefits," he says. "They're seen more positively. Get jobs more easily. Have less difficulty in social situations. They work on their faces, not because they are dissatisfied with their appearance, but because they like it and want to maintain it. They are more invested in health and fitness than the average American. They go to gym, eat a healthy diet." In this context, he adds, a face-lift "is a positive, self-care strategy."

Maintenance. Maintenance. Maintenance. That word had come up continually at my informal cosmetic-surgery discussion group in Scottsdale. Dulcey, one of my guests that night, is by Sarwer's account, a typical face-lift patient. The forty-nine-year-old health-management executive likes her appearance and wants to maintain it. Perfectly turned out in a pink suit that complimented her dark hair and sporting a handsome jeweled brooch, she told the other women in the group why she had a face-lift. "I work out all the time. I eat well. I feel it's all part of fashion," she explained. "But with all that control, I didn't feel like I was all together the way I wanted it to be. Your looks are not necessarily your self-worth, but part of how you think about yourself. I'm not embarrassed about it at all. We're just fighting our heredity along with age. And I plan to do it again in ten years if I need it, or whenever the time comes."

Another guest that night, Cynthia, a fifty-one-year-old retired banker, also talked about maintenance. For her fiftieth birthday, Cynthia gave herself a gift of several cosmetic procedures: upper and lower eyelid-lift, forehead-lift and lower face-lift. "I was preparing my body for the next fifty years because I plan on being around another fifty years. Since I'm divorced, maybe it's a little more important for me to look my best. But I also work out three times a week, and I've done that for ten or fifteen years. So, how my body looks and how my face looks is kind of important to me." And then she used the M word: "It really is maintenance—there was a sagging here," Cynthia said, pointing to her newly crisp jawline, "and I didn't like that. A face-lift doesn't change who you are inside or make you a different person. I wasn't ready to look middle-aged. I wanted to look on the outside the way I felt on the inside. And I'm very energetic and animated."

A friend in Houston, writer Carol Barden, talked to me about maintenance too, although she didn't use the word. She had her face and eyes done when she was only forty-two. "My face wasn't sagging a lot but I was beginning to get a double chin," she said. "I saw a picture of myself in the local paper and didn't like my profile. I decided to do it sooner rather than later. My life wasn't unraveling. I wasn't trying to catch a man. I worked out four and five times a week. I got regular manicures. It seemed like one more thing to do. I don't have a double chin anymore. I feel good when I look in the mirror. I'm glad I did it and I'll do it again. Life goes on."

The Haves vs. the Have-nots-and-Don't-Want-It

There is no more fervent evangelist than a satisfied cosmetic surgery patient. Often, she views the world as one big clinic filled with people waiting for her diagnoses. And when two face-lift veterans get together, it's not long before they are dicing mutual friends who are holdouts.

Six months after her face-lift, "Dawn," the forty-eight-year-old financial consultant we met in chapter two, says she finds herself "looking at people on a bus, on the street, and in restaurants, and thinking, Oh my God, how can she walk around looking like that?" But while Dawn keeps her suggestions to herself, not everyone does.

One New Yorker is a blatant recruiter. She has no hesitation about going up to complete strangers in the gym or at the next table in a restaurant or in a department store, and saying, "You'd look so much prettier with a nose job." Of course, this woman's concern isn't entirely altruistic. She happens to be a professional consultant who gets paid by prospective patients for introducing them to cosmetic surgeons.

Such unsolicited advice doesn't necessarily win friends. One person's new lease on life can be another woman's dispossess notice. Five months after my recent lift, at the annual Valentine's Day party of a friend, designer Joan Vass—another regular at this event—vented to me about plastic-surgery evangelists. After greeting me with a big hello, she scrutinized my face as intensely as a facialist. "You're looking younger. Did you do something new?" she asked, shaking her head in disapproval and launching into her new pet peeve. "The annoying thing about women who have had plastic surgery is, they're always telling you about their surgery and telling you what *you* need and offering to send you to their doctors. Mary McFadden wants me to get my wrinkles filled. I don't want my wrinkles filled," she complains. "You should write about this."

I make it a policy never to volunteer "you-messages": "You ought to have a face-lift." "You ought to have your eyes done." But I may be in the minority. I learned the importance of not making value judgements for other people from Ivo Pitanguy when I made rounds with him in his clinic in Rio. He is adamant that surgeons—or anyone else, for that matter—should not impose their vision on the patient. This was made quite clear during an examination of a sixteen-year-old Brazilian girl with an extremely prominent nose. At first Pitanguy thought she had come to him about her nose. But no. She had uneven breasts. One was large and one was quite small. "The breasts are very important organs," said Pitanguy. "This girl doesn't care about her nose, which is very prominent. She only cares about her breasts. She will have a stigma if she doesn't correct the problem in puberty." After examining the girl, he instructed the nurse to schedule the breast reduction and never mentioned the nose.

The Facilitators

There's a fine line between being a wrinkle policeman and an ombudsman, helping others get the best advice available when they ask for help. I am impressed at how supportive many women can be, without being insulting or autocratic. Rather than being surgery pushers, these women are facilitators.

"Jessica" is such a person. In Hollywood, where "don't ask, don't tell" refers to cosmetic surgery, the forty-two-year-old freelance film editor, broke the code of silence and began talking openly about her assorted surgical alterations. Her candor is a kind of social work. "My way," says Jessica, "of returning the favor others did for me." The women she knows "are all doing preventive stuff. Trying to maintain a look. If they say they're thinking about it, I say, 'I did it and it's great and this is what I've had—eyes, forehead, breasts, hair implants, and teeth capped,' and they look at me in shock. I don't look my age. It's not like I want to shout it to the world. I don't want you to use my real name." But she knows from her own experience, "You need support when you do these things. It is terrifying. You're sitting there waiting for surgery and you feel like an idiot. You're thinking, 'Here I am, perfectly fine, putting myself in an operating room, doing something voluntary and self-centered.' Husbands may be sympathetic," says Jessica, "but they have no idea of what your looks mean to you and how you feel about this 'getting older stuff.' "

Across the country in Louisiana, Georgina, a fifty-ish belle who recently retired from retailing, is another ombudsman. She has found a second calling shepherding buddies through the face-lift rite of passage. Since an eye-lift at age forty-five and a face-lift three years later, Georgina has nudged many friends onto the operating table, even going so far as to drive them the hundred miles to her surgeon's New Orleans clinic.

Georgina tells of meeting a high-school friend in a grocery store. "I hadn't seen her in twenty-five years. I could tell she'd had nothing done." Apparently the old friend could tell that Georgina had had something done, because she told Georgina, "I'm scared to death. I want my eyes done." Taking the cue, Georgina responded, "I've had the whole thing done—eyes, face, neck. Have the whole thing done and you won't talk about it anymore."

I love the idea of women helping friends through this rite of passage. I think of the friend who preceded me into face-lift territory who offered to come to the hospital and put cold compresses on my eyes if I didn't have nurses; the many women I know of who have picked up friends at the hospital and chauffeured them home, staying with them until they could care for themselves; the executive assistant who, to help pay for her lift, rented out her apartment for two weeks and, thus, had no place to recuperate. To her rescue came her boss's lady friend who offered her guestroom for the patient's recuperation.

But I also worry about evangelists who, in their enthusiasm, talk friends into surgery when some people aren't psychologically ready for it.

Take "Dora," recently widowed. Dora called to say she was considering a face-lift and had begun making appointments with surgeons, working down a list given to her by friends. She wanted me to explain why two of the surgeons on her list had separate telephone listings for "Appointments" and for "Nurses." She wondered whether this meant these doctors had a high volume of postoperative problems?

Nurses routinely field patients' lengthy lists of pre- and postoperative questions. It seemed to me that by supplying a separate "nurses" number, the doctors were offering a commendable service. But to Dora, the word "nurses" was frightening. Who knows what memories it conjured in her. This exchange told me that Dora was one of those not yet mentally prepared to go through this. Maybe this friend should tell her so.

Ten

IT'S YOUR DECISION

"The face [is the] focus of anxiety in the aging individual.
Surgery for [it] does not intend to return lost years to the patient, but rather
to make him or her accept his or her biologic age naturally."
—IVO PITANGUY

I had a conversation with my doctor, Dr. Z, the morning after my recent face work. After he inspected his handiwork and decided I was going to turn out fine, he told me the good news: My SMAS has some elasticity left in it yet. "You can have one more lift," he said. For obvious reasons, I haven't shared this news yet with my husband. No need to worry him ahead of time. But I fully expect to exercise the option—although I have no date in mind.

I'm amused at conversations I've had with women who had face-lifts in their forties and fifties but who can't imagine caring about their looks in their sixties. By the time they reach sixty-five, it's possible, of course, that the non-surgical fountain of youth will have arrived. In the next twenty-five years, the face-lift could become obsolete. Work is underway on lasers that will tighten the underlayers of skin without affecting the top ones. Excess internal fat can already be emulsified, externally, using ultrasound. We have every reason to expect ultrasonic technology to make strides—although I worry about reports of skin sensitivity in some patients after ultrasound liposuction. We can also expect a new crop of intelligent vitamins, herbs, and hormones to slow the development of the stigmas of aging—or eliminate them. And, while I refuse to speculate on what beauty miracles the inevitable development of cloning will unleash, it's conceivable that in twenty-five years, instead of going to spas such as The Golden Door for R&R, we'll rejuvenate our sagging skin at gravity-free space resorts.

But one thing that no one expects to change is the desire to look your best. "The nineties may have seen the end of the taboo known as aging," said Rochelle Udell, editor of *Self* in a 1996 speech, "but being beautiful is still the bottom line." And until futuristic beauty treatments are available, surgery is a major option.

The face-lift isn't for everyone. And I'm not advocating it, one way or another, for anyone but myself. It's your decision. A face-lift won't transform you into any of the icons you admire. It won't change your personality. It won't restore your youth.

But it can make you a fresher version of yourself and provide you with a sense of control—and that may give you more confidence. It could give you an advantage or at least level the playing field somewhat in an increasingly competitive job market. But it won't stop the clock from ticking. What a face-lift *will* provide is a lift—an intangible spirit lift.

Does saying "yes" to surgery mean you'll embark on a lifetime process of tinkering, that you'll become a scalpel slave? A recent study estimates that 7 percent of cosmetic surgery patients suffer from this affliction, known as body dismorphic syndrome. The good news is that 93 percent of us *don't* suffer from it. Will we turn into a culture of tightly pulled faces? No more pulled than your favorite TV newscasters. According to my own survey of newsreaders and TV magazine hosts, a large percentage, if not a majority, of them have had some facial surgery—an eye job, a face-lift, neck liposuction, and/or a nose bob—plus regular collagen and Botox shots. And most of these paragons look quite natural.

If a genie could grant me one wish in this regard, it would not be a wish that bags under the eyes and under the chin would be considered beautiful. My wish would be that the influentials, those paragons whose looks define the standards of appearance in our culture, would stand up and give us a count of their facial surgeries. After all, when the busiest plastic surgeon in New York has a one-year waiting list for consultations and those trying to make appointments with a celebrated cosmetic dermatologist must wait months—doesn't that tell us something about the rampant popularity of cosmetic procedures?

Revisiting the diary I kept of my recent operation, I wouldn't call the experience a breeze. Part of the problem was impatience—expecting to be presentable too soon. That puts enormous stress on the already stressed postoperative patient. The other stress was my late-life nose change. I learned that even the slightest change to this feature takes getting used to and can be unsettling to one's family. In retrospect, all the Sturm and Drang over my nose seemed astonishing when I stumbled, the other day, on a snapshot taken three months after the recent nose/brow/lift. It is probably the most flattering picture I've taken in a decade. At last, a picture of myself I didn't want to tear up. Why didn't I realize it at the time?

As I write this, I am days away from a major birthday: "the big seven-oh," I call it, proudly, no longer refusing to say the loathsome word that once marked a woman as not just over-the-hill, but over the mountain. I can deal with it. Call me a "woman of a certain age" but don't call me a "golden ager." I am working and have no plans to stop. My facework has helped me look the way I feel—not any specific numeric age, but rather young-old or vitally mature. I also confess, I have no political objection to the birthday card I've received from my four- and five-year-old grandchildren: a blond Barbie dressed for a prom. Their mother, one of my stepdaughters, tells me, "They picked it themselves. They don't see you as a granny or a bunch of dried flowers."

I've been through it all: the interior dialogue to justify the surgeries, the dilemma of choosing a doctor, the anxiety about the outcome, the guilt, the fear of unexpected consequences, the discomfort, the temporary numbness, the few weeks of downtime, the longer period of self-scrutiny, the panic when I thought there would be a small scar on my lip, the relief when there wasn't, the cost, the sympathetic glances and averted eyes that told me how swollen I was in the beginning, the subsequent expressions of approval from those who mattered to me, and the few snide remarks that indicated jealousy, perhaps, or disdain.

Was it all worth it? Unquestionably, yes. Would I recommend it to friends? Absolutely, as long as they go into it knowing it's not makeup—

it's surgery. Would I do it again? Yes, but with one caveat: knowing what I do now, I would put a little more time between multiple-procedure surgery and my coming out.

The hardest thing about my own face-lift, oddly, has been writing about it. It dawned on me by the time I was well into this project, and loathe to abandon it, that my work might ultimately be judged on what people thought of my face. And, sad to say, two face-lifts, a brow-lift, and a nose job have yet to cure me of my own basic reticence in that department. But, then, the surgery wasn't intended to make me into a model or an icon. I just wanted to be a fresher more confident version of myself.

You want to know what a face-lift will do for you? If you have realistic expectations, it could make you happier than you will ever admit to anyone. Will it change your life? Doubtful. It changed mine because I made a career of writing about plastic surgery, and that's not exactly an option for everyone. But it has also made me more optimistic—dare I say, happy. One reason for this is that my friends are happy for me. It seems that my new face gives them hope and the optimism ricochets. Will it make you a better person? Probably not, although I have become much more understanding of the importance of the face in social relations after seeing one after another self-assured, intelligent, resourceful, powerful woman approach me in a tailspin over her loss of face. Like it or not, fair or unfair, I am—in addition to many other things that define me: intelligence, personality, character, role—my face. You are your face. Change it, ignore it, restore it, let it go, fix it up—it will affect the way others see you. And the way you see yourself. It's your choice and there is no right answer.

CHECK IT OUT

Cosmetic surgery can't be returned for credit like a cosmetic that irritates your face. Validating the quality of the facility where the surgery will take place and looking into the credentials of the person performing the operation—and giving anesthesia—won't guarantee a perfect result, but it will improve the odds. Prospective patients are admonished, over and over again, "do your homework," but how? We used to go to our family doctors for trustworthy referrals. But today, the secretary at an H.M.O. may have replaced the general practitioner who knows you intimately. The onus now is on the patient to do the research. But the sources of information are obscure. We have been raised to respect doctors, but it isn't rude to ask them about their credentials or how many times they have done the procedure in question. Price shouldn't be the only determinant. (If you can't afford the procedures you want, you might consider contacting the plastic surgery department or ear, nose, and throat department of a local university hospital and inquire if volunteers are needed for cosmetic surgical studies or demonstrations.)

Here is a short list of organizations that can supply information on anesthesia; a doctor's training and credentials; and the accreditation of a non-hospital operation room—or refer you to qualified specialists in your geographical area. It's your only face, and good information is the best foundation for any restoration and reconstruction project.

Operating Room Accreditation

Joint Commission for the Accreditation of Healthcare Organizations
One Renaissance Boulevard
Oakbrook Terrace, IL 60181
Phone: (630) 916-5600
Fax: (630) 792-5005
Web site Address: www.jcaho.org
Callers can confirm a medical or healthcare facility's accreditation status and receive information on accreditation criteria and standards.

Accreditation Association for Ambulatory Health Care
9933 Lawler Avenue
Suite 460
Skokie, IL 60077
Phone: (847) 676-9610
Fax: (847) 676-9628
Callers can confirm a facility's accreditation status and receive information on accreditation standards.

American Association for Accreditation of Ambulatory Surgery Facilities, Inc.
1202 Allanson Road
Mundelein, IL 60060
Phone: (847) 949-6058
Fax: (847) 566-4580
Toll-Free: (888) 545-5222
Web site Address: www.surgeon.org
Telephone referral line to confirm a facility's accreditation status and check a doctor's board certification.

Medical Credentials and Board Certification

American Medical Association
515 N. State Street
Chicago, IL 60610
Phone: (312) 464-5000
Fax: (312) 464-4184
Web site Address: www.ama-assn.org
Physician Data Licensing Area
(312) 464-6201
Callers can confirm that a doctor is a member and holds a valid medical license.

American Board of Medical Specialties
1007 Church Street
Suite 404
Evanston, IL 60201
Phone: (847) 491-9091
Fax: (847) 328-3596
Toll-Free: (800) 776-2378
Web site Address: www.abms.org/abms
Telephone referral line to confirm a doctor's board certification.

American Board of Medical Specialties

24 MEMBER CERTIFYING BOARDS

American Board of Allergy and Immunology
American Board of Anesthesiology
American Board of Colon and Rectal Surgery
American Board of Dermatology
American Board of Emergency Medicine
American Board of Family Practice

American Board of Internal Medicine
American Board of Medical Genetics
American Board of Neurological Surgery
American Board of Nuclear Medicine
American Board of Obstetrics and Gynecology
American Board of Ophthalmology
American Board of Orthopaedic Surgery
American Board of Otolaryngology
American Board of Pathology
American Board of Pediatrics
American Board of Physical Medicine and Rehabilitation
American Board of Plastic Surgery
American Board of Preventive Medicine
American Board of Psychiatry and Neurology
American Board of Radiology
American Board of Surgery
American Board of Thoracic Surgery
American Board of Urology

American College of Surgeons
633 N. St. Clair Street
Chicago, IL 60611
Phone: (312) 202-5000
Fax: (312) 202-5001
Web site Address: www.facs.org
Callers can confirm that a doctor is a member and receive information on fourteen clinical procedures as well as the socioeconomic and legal aspects of surgery.

American Board of Plastic Surgery
Seven Penn Center, Suite 400
1635 Market Street
Philadelphia, PA 19103-2204
Phone: (215) 587-9322
Fax: (215) 587-9622
Web site Address: abpsphl@p3.net
Callers can confirm that a doctor is a board-certified plastic surgeon.

Specialty Educational Associations

CHECK CREDENTIALS AND GET REFERRALS

American Society for Aesthetic Plastic Surgery
36 W. 44th Street, Suite 630
New York, NY 10036

Phone: (212) 921-0500
Fax: (212) 921-0011
Web site Address: www.surgery.org
Cosmetic Plastic Surgery Referral Line
Phone: (888) 272-7711
Telephone referral line for board-certified plastic surgeons in your geographical area; callers can receive information on aesthetic plastic surgical techniques.

American Society of Plastic and Reconstructive Surgeons
444 E. Algonquin Road
Arlington Heights, IL 60005
Phone: (847) 228-9900
Fax: (847) 228-9131
Web site Address: www.plasticsurgery.org
Plastic Surgery Referral Service
Phone: (800) 364-6464
Telephone referral line for board-certified plastic surgeons in your geographical area.

American Association of Facial Plastic and Reconstructive Surgeons
310 S. Henry Street
Alexandria, VA 22314
Phone: (703) 299-9291
Fax: (703) 299-8898
Web site Address: www.facial-plastic-surgery.org
Toll-Free: (800) 332-3223
Telephone referral line for board-certified dermatologists, otolaryngologists, and plastic surgeons in your geographical area.

American Society for Dermatologic Surgery
930 N. Meacham Road
Schaumburg, IL 60173
Phone: (800) 441-2737
Fax: (847) 330-1090
Web site Address: www.asds-net.org
Callers can confirm that a doctor is a member and receive information on dermatologic surgical procedures.

American Society for Laser Medicine and Surgery
2404 Stewart Square
Wausau, WI 54401
Phone: (715) 845-9283
Fax: (715) 848-2493
Web site Address: www.aslms.org
Callers can confirm that a doctor is a member and receive referrals to doctors in their geographical area.

Anesthesia Information

American Society of Anesthesiologists
520 N. Northwest Highway
Park Ridge, IL 60068
Phone: (847) 825-5586
Fax: (847) 825-1692
Web site Address: www.asahq.org
Callers can confirm that a doctor is board-certified and receive information on anesthesia techniques.

Anesthesia Patient Safety Foundation
Phone: (412) 281-9484
Open Monday, Tuesday, and Thursday.

When in Doubt

The following resources have valuable up-to-date information on drug side effects, interactions, and dosing schedules.

BOOKS

Complete Drug Reference: 1998. United States Pharmacopoeia, Consumer Reports Books, 1997.

Deadly Drug Interactions: The People's Pharmacy Guide. Joe Graedon and Teresa Graedon, Ph.D., St. Martin's Griffin, 1997.

The Pill Book. 7th ed., Harold M. Silverman and Ian Ginsberg, editors, Bantam Books, 1996.

WEB SITES

Healthtouch
www.healthtouch.com

Institute for Safe Medication Practices
www.ismp.org

Pharmaceutical Information Network
www.pharminfo.com

U.S. Food and Drug Administration
www.fda.gov

U.S. Pharmacopoeia
www.usp.org

ACKNOWLEDGMENTS

When my husband asked me, in 1996, where I wanted to go to celebrate our twenty-fifth anniversary, I said "Venice." It's a city I love, but it's also not that far from Bologna, and I was determined, before this book was finished, to see the anatomy theater of Gaspare Tagliacozzi—the sixteenth-century anatomist who is considered the grandfather of plastic surgery. He rebuilt noses for nobels and peasants who lost them to disease, punishment, or sword fights. But where exactly in Bologna was I headed? Several calls and faxes to a tourist office and to the University of Bologna yielded no addresses. Then Roberta Libanore at Condé Nast's office in Milan came to the rescue. She found Dr. Licio Baroncini, a plastic and reconstructive surgeon, whose office in Bologna is located, coincidentally, on via Tagliacozzi, and Dr. Baroncini offered not just directions, but to be my tour guide. Thus, on a chilly day at the end of March, when my husband and I drove into Bologna, Dr. Baroncini was waiting patiently for us in the town square. For no reward other than pride in his city's heritage and love of history, he devoted his day to giving us—total strangers—a tour of the Tagliacozzi landmarks. I followed him up a narrow staircase in the stacks of a medical library, and down a long hall to see the only two paintings in existence of the legendary doctor. But the highlight of the tour was the life-size statue of Tagliacozzi holding a severed nose in his hand. It occupies a gold-leafed niche in the wood-paneled anatomy theater in Bologna's Hospitale del Mortes, built centuries ago over Bologna's catacombs in the Old City area and restored after World War II.

Dr. Baroncini's graciousness is typical of the help I have received from strangers, colleagues, and friends in preparing this book.

Allure has, in a sense, sent me to graduate school on this subject, publishing, to date, seventeen of my articles on plastic and cosmetic surgery and sending me on assignments and to plastic surgery conferences all over the U.S. and, occasionally, abroad. *Allure's* editor-in-chief, Linda Wells, realized before I did how fascinated and conflicted we all are on this subject, and not only has she sponsored my education, she suggested many story ideas and has been a responsive sounding board and ally. My first article on the topic, "Shopping for a Face-lift," was edited with sensitivity by Susan Roy (who was instrumental in my association with the magazine). When it was published, Sue's husband Randy Rothenberg, a fellow journalist, insisted "There's a book in this" and outlined how it should be written. It took me a few years to see the light.

I.C.M.'s Amanda Urban, my literary agent, helped me focus the concept and found exactly the right person to publish the book—Wendy Wolf, an editor who understands ambivalence about appearance issues first-hand. She jokes that she needs "anesthesia for a haircut." After coming up with the title, she teased this book out of me with smart advice and stern affection. Her most appreciated editorial decision was not asking me to supply my before and after pictures. She understood better than I what the tone should be and when I finally hit the right note, she left a message on my machine: "You've found your voice, keep going." I replayed it every day for months before erasing it.

Several other editors have left their marks on this text. They are the former and current *Allure* editors who have sharpened my prose and point of view in one or another of my plastic surgery articles (some of which are quoted or referenced in this work): besides Susan Roy, they are Paula Chin, Lucy Danziger, David DeNicolo, Carol Kramer, Dianne Partie Lange, Martha McCully, Katherine Russell Rich, Ilene Rosenzweig, Mary Turner, and the inimitable Tom Prince. Larry Karol arranged the ways and the means. Eileen Baum has verified virtually every word I've written on this subject for the magazine—and has done the same for this volume. Her marathon labor on this book, every night after doing her day job, for nearly a month, was beyond the call. Attorneys Stanley Rothenberg, Jerry Birenz, Richard Constantine, Randy Dryer, and Viking's counsel, Maura Wogan, have coached me, over the years, on the art of being accurate without being harmful. But, inevitably, there will be mistakes or misinterpretations of data and I take full responsibility for them.

Those at Viking who have helped this book into the world include Nelly Bly, Reeve Chace, Jennifer Kobylarz, Paul Buckley, Barbara Grossman, Patti Kelly, and Breene Farrington.

I am not a doctor. Grasping the theory and technique of plastic surgery well enough to explain it has been a constant effort. Sam Kron was my first surgery instructor. Several plastic surgeons have (with their patients' approval) allowed me to watch operations, including Sherrell Aston, Sam Hamra, Vladimir Mitz, Ivo Pitanguy, and Gerald Pitman, and dermatologist Jeffrey Dover.

In the history department, Hale Tolleth, Phillip Casson, Gustavo Colon, Robert Goldwyn, Willard Marmelzat, and Ralph Millard lent books, sent articles, and made introductions. Blair O. Rogers, perhaps the pre-eminent historian on cosmetic surgery, has been generous with his time, advice, and reprints. There is no way I could have written this without reading his papers.

Scores of M.D.s (in addition to those mentioned above) have spent hours on the phone and in person talking to me about various issues, from Hollywood history to face-lifting techniques. They include Adrien Aiache, Bernard Alpert, Donald Altman, Vijay Anand, Gaspar Anastasi, Richard Aronsohn, Daniel Baker, Thomas Baker, Fritz Barton, Jr., Bradley Bengtson, Robert Bernard, T. George Brennan, Garry Brody, Stafford Broumand, Jay Burns, Henry Steve Byrd, James Carraway, Salvador Castanares, Bruce Connell, Eugene Courtiss, Rollin Daniel, Franklin DiSpaltro, Richard Ellenbogen, Stephen Fagien, Joel Feldman, Robert Flowers, Garth Fisher, Jack Fisher, Peter Bela Fodor, Craig Foster, Jack Friedland, Simon Fredricks, Stephen Genender, Alan Gold, Frederic Grazer, A. Richard Grossman, John Grossman, Jack Gunter, Edward Guy, Roxanne Guy, Robert Hamas, Barbara Hayden, David Hidalgo, Steven Hoefflin, Ronald Iverson, Glenn Jelcks, Mark Jewell, Henry Kawamoto, Frank Kamer, Michael Kane, Bernard Kaye, Brian Kinney, Robert Kotler, Val Lambros, Edward Lamont, Norman Leaf, Richard Leinhardt, Mark Lemmon, Richard Lisman, Paul Lorenc, Timothy Marten, Alan Matarasso, G. Patrick Maxwell, Joseph McCarthy, Peter McKinney, Timothy Miller, John Owsley, Morey Parkes, Malcolm Paul, Oscar Ramirez, Thomas Rees, Brunno Ristow, Rod Rohrich, Gary Rosenberg, Frank Ryan, Kenneth Salyer, Bernard Sarnat, Lawrence Seifert, Norman Schorr, Daniel Shapiro, Jack Sheen, Robert Singer, James Smith, Wendell Smoot, III, Ewaldo Souza Pinto,

James Stuzin, Nicholas Tabbal, Gary Tearston, John Tebbetts, Bahman Teimourian, Stephen Teitelbaum, Edward Terino, Dennis Thompson, Edward Truppman, Charles Vinnik, James Wells, Linton Whitaker, Tolbert Wilkinson, John Williams, Donald Wood-Smith, John Yousif, Harvey Zarem, Barry Zide, and Mark Zukowski.

Tina Alster, Frederic Brandt, Jay Burns, Jean Carruthers, Alistair Carruthers, Anita Cela, Richard Fitzpatrick, Ellen Gendler, Roy Geronemus, Richard Glogau, Richard Gregory, Melanie Grossman, Arnold Klein, Seth Matarasso, Ronald Moy, Rhoda Narins, Thomas Roberts, III, Jack Rozen, Phillip Stone, Mark Rubin, and Patricia Wexler (all M.D.s) have shared their knowledge in skin matters. Aestheticians Christina Carlino, Jacqueline Stallone, Jacque Thomas, Vera Brown, and Helena Ballas expanded my knowledge of the history of skin peeling. I am indebted to Dr. Terino for introducing me to the late Arthur Gradé, the legendary lay peeler. Robert Goldwyn has been my guru on the doctor-patient relationship; Mark Gorney and Charles O'Brien on patient dissatisfaction; Michael McGuire, Daniel Morello, Gustavo Colon, and Edward Truppman on office accreditation. Alan Matarasso has helped me understand complications. L. David Silver and Tom Nyberg gave me a crash course in anesthesia. Nurses Peggy Broderick, Donna Phillips, Margie Stemberger, and recovery house owner Nola Rocco helped me fine-tune my knowledge of postoperative recovery.

Sherrell Aston read this book for technical accuracy, always respecting my right to my opinions—even though he may have disagreed. I am deeply indebted to him, but, again, any inaccuracies are my own.

Much of my library research was done at the New York Academy of Medicine Library, the New York Public Library (with special assistance from its NY Public Library Express research service), and at the library of Manhattan Eye, Ear & Throat Hospital (MEETH). A special thanks to Dede Silverston, director of MEETH's library, who supplied me with endless reference papers, ordered in rare books from obscure libraries—and taught me to use the Internet for scientific research. Thanks also to George Feifer, a dedicated volunteer in MEETH's library. On the trail of Cleopatra's image I was guided by Marsha Hill, associate curator in the department of Egyptian Art at the Metropolitan Museum of Art, and Sara Fitzsimmons at The Brooklyn Museum.

Harvard's Frances A. Countway Library is the official archive of plastic surgery in the U.S. and a rich resource. I am indebted to librarian Madeleine Mullin for her knowledgeable and intuitive assistance—and her hospitality.

Through the years, I have been helped immeasurably in my understanding of this subject by the staff members of several professional organizations—notably Elizabeth Sadati and, more recently, Barbara Callas of The American Society for Aesthetic Plastic Surgery, and Phil Saigh, Nancy Ryan, and Beverly Jones of the American Society of Plastic and Reconstructive Surgeons. But no one was as helpful as Nancy Kobus, the former ASAPS media coordinator. Nancy came through, once again, by helping me compile and check the Source Directory at the end of this book.

Andrea Miller accurately typed hours of discussion group transcripts; Bruce Stark kept my computers from crashing. Ed Shanahan helped me organize, edit, and re-edit mountains of first-draft text into a coherent final draft, and input and edited almost four hundred end notes (thank you Barbara Graustark for introducing us). Jeffries Blackerby, Skye Donald, Eleni Gage, Jane Havsy, and Lisa Krohn helped with research and organization.

I have also had help from physician e-mail pals around the world: Luiz Toledo (and his wife Kate) in São Paulo; Ivo Pitanguy in Rio de Janeiro; Claude Perpere in

Marseilles who helped me pin down details about doctors Noël, Dujarier, and Joseph. My Paris correspondents have been doctors Gilbert Aiach, Eric Auclair, Yves-Gérard Illouz, Patrick Knipper, Daniel Marchac, Vladimir Mitz, and Dominick Rheims. Noreen Hall ran interference and translated.

In private conversations and in group discussions, dozens of consumers—women and men—shared their personal feelings and stories. I promised them anonymity so I can't thank them by name—but this book is their story as much as mine. Others who have added to the texture of this book, or helped me in one way or another are Mouna Al-Ayoub, Drs. Magdalena and Kalman Berenyi, Dr. Patricia Allen, Martha Barnette, Walter Bernard, Rachel Bolton of Hallmark Cards, Mario Buatta, Barbara Caplan of Yankelovich Partners, Kimberly Callet, Myron Chin, Judy Cohen, Norma Collier, Norman Covert of Fort Deitrick, Gladys Cutler, Rosemary Eckersly, Barbara and Stanley Feldman, Frederic Fekkai, Barbara Flood, Lisa Gabor, Sandy Golinkin, Nina Griscom, Stephen Gullo, Constance Hartnett, Gale Hayman, Sandy Hill, Robin Hodes, Wendy Holden, Robert Woodfin Jones, Janet Kardon, Kasumi Kasai, Susan Kelleher, Barbara Kling, Ted Kruckel, Francine Leinhardt, Kathy Leventhal, Simone Levitt, Wendy Lewis, Judy Licht, Bari Lynn, Masha Magaloff, Pablo Manzoni, Diana McLellen, Polly Allen Mellen, Nolan Miller, John Montorio, Michele de Monseras, Lois Morris, Victoria Oberfeld, Gloria Parkes, David Peretz, Ron Prince, Joan Rackmil, Joanna Rice, Margot Rogoff, Ruth Kauders Rothchild, Blair Sabol, Michael Sands, Ralph Schlissberg, Fred Schwartz, Jane Singer, Suzanne Slesin, Candy Spelling, Michael Steinberg, Tricia Trask O'Leary, Lindsy Van Gelder, Maria Goulart Viveiros, Sean Young, Janet Zebooker, the research departments at the *Ladies Home Journal* and Condé Nast Publications. I'm sure this list is incomplete.

Teri Agins, Meg Cox, Alan Halpern, Dianne Lange, and Lee Whittington read early drafts and gave encouragement. Stuart Ewen, Jacque Lynn Foltyn, Arthur Frank, Grant McCracken, Frances Cooke Macgregor, Gail Sheehy, Michael Solomon, and Brian Turner helped me think about the social psychology of the subject. Clay Felker has been a mentor and cheerleader, as was the late Lucy Kroll. Writing books—especially one with so much technical information—is difficult, but the work was a pleasure because of the interaction with so many generous professionals. Each morning, it was exciting to see what missive was waiting for me on my fax machine or in e-mail from far-flung places. My life has been enriched by these connections.

Writers' families are used to being neglected. My family had a double burden. With fingers crossed that all would go well medically, my gang cringed through my two bouts of face work—and then got short shrift for the two years it took me to write this memoir. My sincere thanks to my mother Rose Feldman, and my brood: Daniel Kron, Geane Brito, Peter McGratten, Jonathan Marder, Jane Marder, Matthew Martin, Susan Zelouf, and Dr. David Zelouf—who was always there to answer medical questions. But most of all, I want to thank "J"—my husband Jerry Marder—who endured all of the above plus the indignity of having his frank observations of my post-operative progress recorded. I apologize if I have embarrassed him. If I were to reveal how many ways he helped me—in spite of his reluctance to have me nose around the subject—I would embarrass him more. He is the proverbial man you can lean on.

There is only one other person to thank, and that is Dr. Z (a made-up initial), the surgeon who did my two lifts. There are many talented and caring plastic surgeons around the world and I feel terribly lucky to have found one of them.

NOTES

CHAPTER ONE: HOW I GOT THIS FACE

page 1: "There are only two things worth talking about": Gail Sheehy, *The Silent Passage: Menopause* (New York: Random House, 1991, 1992), p. 3.

page 4: "the piece ran a few months later": Anonymous, "Shopping for a New Face," *Allure*, August 1992, pp. 118–123, 131.

page 4: "growing old disgracefully": term coined by Salman Rushdie in "India at Five-O," *Time*, August 11, 1997, p. 40.

page 5: "the plastic-surgery star system": Joan Kron, "The Nip-and-Tuck Career of Ivo Pitanguy," *Allure*, September 1994, pp. 194–199, 230–231.

page 5: "Patient who murdered her plastic surgeon": Joan Kron, "Appointment with Death," *Allure*, February 1994, pp. 102–105, 147.

page 5: "cosmetic surgery's most visible consumer": Joan Kron, "The Man in the Mirror: Doctors Analyze the Faces of Michael Jackson," *Allure*, January 1996, pp. 116–119, 139, 140.

page 5: " 'the Twins Study' ": Joan Kron, "Dueling Face-Lifts," *Allure*, August 1996, pp. 82, 84, 86, 99.

page 6: "Steinem had an eye-lift": Gloria Steinem, *Revolution from Within: A Book of Self-Esteem* (Boston: Little Brown, 1992), p. 241.

page 6: "Brown, meanwhile, favors it wholeheartedly": Nancy Lloyd, "Helen Gurley Brown: Still the Same ol' Tease," *Modern Maturity*, May–June 1997, pp. 54–59. (When asked about cosmetic surgery, Brown said, "My God, it's out there, it's wonderful, it's better than ever.")

page 6: "Upper eye-lifts were performed": Blair O. Rogers, M.D., "History of Oculoplastic Surgery," *Aesthetic Plastic Surgery*, 1988, Vol 12: pp. 129–152. (Quoted in Peter A. Adamson and Mary Lynn Moran, "Historical Trends in Surgery for the Aging Face," *Facial Plastic Surgery*, Vol 9, No. 2, April 1993, pp. 133–142.)

page 7: "A recipe, written in hieroglyphs": James Henry Breasted, *The Edwin Smith Surgical Papyrus* (Chicago: University of Chicago Press, 1930, vol. 1), pp. 506–507.

page 7: "in her old age, outlawed looking glasses": Maggie Angeloglou, *A History of Makeup* (Great Britain: The Macmillan Company, 1970), p. 52.

page 7: "A woman's current life expectancy": Jane E. Brody, "Estrogen after menopause? A tough dilemma," *The New York Times*, August 20, 1997, p. C8.

page 8: "Friends can be a great support": James May, Jr., "Preoperative and Postoperative Care for Patients Undergoing Blepharoplasty and Face Lift," *Aesthetic Surgery Journal*, May/June, 1997, pp. 192–194.

CHAPTER TWO: IT'S NOT NICE TO FOOL MOTHER NATURE

page 9: "[America] was founded on the revolutionary principle": Gilbert Seldes, *The Great Audience* (New York: The Viking Press, 1950). (Quoted in Ann Douglas, *Terrible Honesty: Mongrel Manhattan in the 1920s* [New York: Farrar, Straus and Giroux, 1995], p. 448.)

page 9: "one of the 90,000 or so women": Source: "ASAPS 1997 Statistics on Cosmetic Surgery" (New York: American Society for Aesthetic Plastic Surgery, 1998).

page 10: "35 percent . . . say they'd never have one again": Thomas L. Roberts, III, M.D. and Laura B. Ellis, M.D. "In Pursuit of Optimal Rejuvenation of the Forehead: Endoscopic Browlift with Simultaneous CO_2 Laser Resurfacing," *Plastic & Reconstructive Surgery*, Vol. 101, April 1998. (See Table 3: Patient Satisfaction: 88.5 percent had a pleasing result, but only 65 percent would do it again, while of the patients who had an endoscopic lift plus laser resurfacing, 97 percent would do it again.)

page 11: "If you change one feature": Author's interview with Barry Zide, M.D., October 1996.

page 11: "One sign of post-modern society": Author's interview with Canadian anthropologist Grant McCracken, January 1993.

page 12: "hanging out at tattoo parlors": Clinton R. Sanders, *Customizing the Body: The Art and Culture of Tattooing* (Philadelphia: Temple University Press, 1989).

page 12: "Moore . . . who disguised herself": Mike Featherstone and Mike Hepworth, "The Mask of Ageing and the Postmodern Life Course," 1989. (In M. Featherstone, M. Hepworth, and B. Turner, *The Body: Social Process and Cultural Theory* [London: Sage Publications, 1991], pp. 377–379.)

page 12: " 'a beautiful visage often plays a role' ": Alex Kuczynski, "Concierge to the Literary Pack," *The New York Times*, Sunday Styles, January 11, 1998, Section 9, pp. 1 (Col 1), 6.; *see also* Frank Rich, "Star of the Month Club," *The New York Times*, March 23, 1997, p. 15. (Rich talks about "the Hollywoodization of publishing" with its "growing emphasis on writers with movie-star looks.")

page 14: "cosmetic surgery 'is not ... imposed upon women' ": Kathy Davis, *Reshaping the Female Body: The Dilemma of Cosmetic Surgery* (New York: Routledge, 1995), p. 5. This is a study of the sociology of cosmetic surgery and the meaning of appearance in women's lives (see also Kathy Davis, "Remaking the She-Devil: A Critical Look at Feminist Approaches to Beauty," *Hypatia* Vol. 6, No. 2, Summer 1991, pp. 21–43).

page 15: "erase signs of aging ... move the recipient": Clinton R. Sanders, *Customizing the Body: The Art and Culture of Tattooing* (Philadelphia: Temple University Press, 1989), p. 7.

page 16: "With over four million baby boomers turning forty every year": Jennifer Cheeseman Day, *Population Projections of the United States by Age, Sex, Race, and Hispanic Origin: 1995 to 2050*, U.S. Bureau of the Census, Current Population Reports (Washington, D.C.: U.S. Government Printing Office, 1996).

page 16: "a very long old age": Cynthia Crossen, "Growing Up Goes On and On and On," *The Wall Street Journal*, March 24, 1997, pp. B1, B7.

page 16: "*female* jurors, are unsympathetic": based on author's interviews with Houston plaintiff lawyer Richard Mithoff, who specializes in medical malpractice, February 1994; and Walnut Creek, CA, lawyer Charles O'Brien, a lawyer with the Doctors Company, a major malpractice insurer of plastic surgeons, February 1994. ("Juries, by and large, are receptive to people who had plastic surgery for medical reasons and suffered some kind of injury," says Mithoff. "But they are much *less* receptive to [complaints about] surgery done purely for cosmetic reasons. There are a lot of people who feel that if you go around having surgery on your body just to make yourself feel more beautiful, you deserve what you get." In the jury selection process, says Mithoff, "we try to remind potential jurors that our society, our culture, puts a lot of pressure on young women to look as good as they can." *Women* jurors are particularly tough on cosmetic surgery patients. In preparation for defending against breast-implant litigation in California, O'Brien staged mock trials before five demographically typical juries—"sixty people in all, black, white, wealthy, and poor," he says. The trials showed "men were more sympathetic to women wanting to make themselves more attractive—and women were markedly less so.")

page 16: "waste of social resources": Charles Strouse, "Aged to Imperfection: Plastic Surgery Latest Wrinkle for Boomers," *The Miami Herald*, January 16, 1995, pp. A1, A6. (Quote from Dr. Arthur Caplan, a medical ethicist at the University of Pennsylvania: "There's a real ethical question here of how much of the world's resources should go to making people look better.")

page 17: "an American obsession": Letty Cottin Pogrebin speech, 92nd Street Y, New York, NY, June 3, 1996.

page 17: "The French, once holdouts": Author's correspondence with Docteur Gilbert Aiach, of Paris, April 1998. (Also Laurence Bagot, "Le Business Sulfureux de la Chirurgie Esthétique," *Capital*, June 1996, pp. 110–112, 114.)

page 17: "face-lifts are fattening the bank accounts ...": "In Beirut, it's Beauty and the Bust," Internet report by Reuters, August 12, 1997. (Also Steve Glain, "Cosmetic Surgery Goes Hand in Glove with the New Korea," *The Wall Street Journal*, November 23, 1993, pp. A1, A5; "India Culture: Rich Pursue Physical Perfection," *IPS* News Service [Internet report], October 28, 1996.)

page 17: "It's considered 'permanent makeup' by Venezuela's beauty pageant participants": Report on Venezuelan beauty pageants, *Dateline NBC*, August 13, 1997.

page 17: "the typical Girl from Ipanema averages three beauty surgeries in her lifetime": Author's correspondence with São Paulo plastic surgeon Luiz Toledo, M.D., 1997. (Toledo was quoting figures compiled by the Brazil Society of Plastic Surgery.)

page 17: "concerned with her vanishing looks": Maggie Angeloglou, *A History of Makeup* (New York: The Macmillan Company, 1970), p. 52.

page 18: "Glassner traces twentieth-century self-consciousness to the birth of the printing press": Barry Glassner, *Bodies: Why We Look the Way We Do (and How We Feel About It)* (New York: G.P. Putnam's Sons, 1988), pp. 27–29.

page 18: "self-scrutiny soared": Ibid. p. 28. (According to Glassner, sales of eyeglasses increased "thirtyfold" between 1880 and 1929.)

page 18: "By the end of World War I": Ann Douglas, *Terrible Honesty: Mongrel Manhattan in the 1920s* (New York: Farrar, Straus & Giroux, 1995), p. 190.

page 18: "The artillery caused wounds": John Staige Davis, "Plastic Surgery in World War I and in World War II," Presidential address to the American Association of Plastic Sugeons, Toronto, Can., June 3, 1946.

page 18: "Before the war there was only one": Ibid.

page 19: "High Definition Television . . . will raise even higher": Raymond Sokolov, "The Best TV Picture You've Never Seen," *The Wall Street Journal*, March 20, 1997, p. A14.

page 20: "People often opt for cosmetic changes": John W. Schouten, "Selves in Transition: Symbolic Consumption in Personal Rites of Passage and Identity Reconstruction," *Journal of Consumer Research* (Chicago: University of Chicago Press, March 1991, Volume 17, No. 4), pp. 412–425.

page 20: "life expectancy . . . in 1994 . . . was 75.7 years": Gina Kolata, "Model Shows How Medical Changes Let Population Surge," *The New York Times*, January 7, 1997, p. C3.

page 20: " 'no matter how secure you feel' ": Hal Lancaster, "Managing Your Career: Why Retire at All? Here's How to Launch a Postcareer Career," *The Wall Street Journal*, August 5, 1997, p. B1.

page 20: "pulchritude [pays] handsomely": C.M. Bosman, G. Pfann, J.E. Biddle, D.S. Hamermesh, "Business Success and Businesses' Beauty Capital," National Bureau of Economic Research, Working Paper No. 6083, July 1, 1997.

page 21: "In previous centuries, the individual was embedded": Author's interview with Grant McCracken, August 1996.

page 21: "One IBM executive underwent cosmetic surgery": Pete Barlas, "Many Go Under the Knife to Stay on Top of Careers," *San Jose and Silicon Valley Business Journal*, July 15–21, 1996, pp. 1B, 10B.

page 21: " 'At my age, you become more of a spokesperson' ": "Page Six," *New York Post*, September 17, 1996.

page 21: "a 50-percent increase in the number of patients undergoing wrinkle-diminishing chemical peels": conclusion based on comparison of the national procedural totals in "1994 Plastic Surgery Statistics" with "1996 Plastic Surgery Statistics" compiled by the American Society of Plastic and Reconstructive Surgeons (ASPRS), Arlington Heights, IL 60005-4664.

page 22: "For the young at heart who wish they had a face to go with it": Advertisement for Constructive Surgery, *New York*, March 31, 1997, p. 6.

CHAPTER THREE: LOSING FACE

page 23: "I used to think cosmetic surgery was stupid. . . . And now I don't": Barbara and Jim Dale, *Dale Cards*, B-084153, RPG, Inc. Chicago, IL.

page 24: "who feels trapped in a body": Kathy Davis, *Reshaping the Female Body: The Dilemma of Cosmetic Surgery* (New York: Routledge, 1995).

page 25: "the idea of not being this way": *Daily Express*, June 8, 1992. (Quoted in Efrat Tseelon, *The Masque of Femininity: The Presentation of Woman in Everyday Life* [London: Sage, 1995], p. 80.)

page 25: "more chins than the Hong Kong phone book?": Diana McLellan, "Young Again!" *Washingtonian*, September 1989, pp. 160–172.

page 25: "I think it is helpful for women to see mature images": Marion Hume, "The Cat in the Hat," *The Independent on Sunday*, September 19, 1993, pp. 18–21. (Meisel was born in 1954.)

page 25: "young or dead": Ann Douglas, *Terrible Honesty: Mongrel Manhattan in the 1920s*, (New York: Farrar, Straus & Giroux, 1995), p. 473.

page 25: "You think of him as *being* an ancestor": *The Tonight Show with Jay Leno*, September 13, 1996.

page 26: " 'old boiler, old trout' ": Allison Pearson, "Letter From London: Love in a Cold Climate," *The New Yorker*, August 25/September 1, 1997, pp. 124–133.

page 26: "She died young and beautiful still.": Liz Smith with Dennis Ferrara, "England Has Lost It's Only Real Queen," *New York Post*, September 1, 1997, p. 12.

page 26: "wrinkles and red eyes mark an old woman": "Elderly Women Face Rampant Murder in Tanzania" (interview with Ms. Mary Nagu, the Minister for Social Development, Women and Children; and with Mwanza, AAANA, Regional Commissioner Major General James Lubanga), Internet report from All Africa Press Service, February 9, 1998, 20:34:00.

page 26: " 'make you believe in love' ": Online commentary by "a reader," *The Bridges of Madison County* discussion site, Amazon.com, September 28, 1996.

page 26: "divorced his fifty-six-year-old wife' ": Richard Johnson, "Page Six: Burnt Bridges," *New York Post*, October 2, 1997, p. 8.

page 26: "We were once obliged": Grant McCracken, *Plenitude: Culture by Commotion* (Toronto: Periph.: Fluide, 1997), p. 21.

page 26: "discourse of justification": Kathy Davis, *Reshaping the Female Body: The Dilemma of Cosmetic Surgery* (New York: Routledge, 1995), p. 4.

page 26: "builds her case": Ibid., pp. 125–126.

page 27: " 'never fully incorporated' ": John M. Goin, M.D., and Marcia K. Goin, Ph.D., "Psychological Aspects of Aesthetic Plastic Surgery," in John R. Lewis, Jr., M.D., ed. *The Art of Aesthetic Plastic Surgery* (Boston: Little, Brown and Company, 1989), pp. 39–47.

page 27: "started sleeping on her back": Elizabeth Snead, "Face to Face with Surgery: A Few Bumps on N.C. Woman's Road to Recovery," *USA Today*, July 1, 1996, p. 6D.

page 27: "foolish ploy to try to reverse time": Bernice Kanner, "Face to Face: One Woman's Uplifting Story," *New York*, June 3, 1991, pp. 36–39.

page 28: " 'tell you they want to grow old gracefully' ": Thomas D. Rees, M.D., *More Than Just a Pretty Face: How Cosmetic Surgery Can Improve Your Looks and Your Life* (Boston: Little, Brown, and Company, 1987), p. 7.

page 30: "award-winning series on aging": Penny Crone, *The Fountain of Youth* (New York: Fox TV), May 1–6, 1995.

page 31: " 'went into a tailspin' ": Letty Cottin Pogrebin, *Getting Over Getting Older* (Boston: Little, Brown and Company, 1996), pp. 132–133.

page 32: "meddling with the handiwork of God": Martha Teach Gnudi and Jerome Pierce Webster, *The Life and Times of Gaspare Tagliacozzi, Surgeon of Bologna* (New York: Herbert Reichner, 1950), p. 304.

page 32: "buried in hallowed ground": Maxwell Maltz, M.D., *Evolution of Plastic Surgery* (New York: Froben, 1946), p. 164.

page 33: " 'terminal ugliness' ": Naomi Wolf, *The Beauty Myth* (London: Chatto & Windus, 1990), p. 195.

page 33: " 'change the rules' ": Ibid., p. 239.

page 33: "her own eyelid operation": Gloria Steinem, *Revolution from Within: A Book of Self-Esteem* (Boston: Little, Brown and Company, 1992), pp. 239, 241.

page 33: " 'Should I stand for the right to have wrinkles?' ": Pamela Kruger, *Working Woman,* July 1994, pp. 55–60, 84, 87.

page 34: " 'Damnation was the punishment' ": Maggie Angeloglou, *A History of Makeup* (New York: The Macmillan Company, 1970), p. 52.

page 34: "first plastic-surgery shopping story": Ethel Lloyd Patterson, "Face Value: Why Grow Old," *Ladies Home Journal,* September 1922, pp. 28, 159. (According to the Oxford English Dictionary, linguists first noticed the term face-lift in F. Courtenay's 1922 book, *Physical Beauty,* ix. 57: "the face-raising or face-lifting process which does away with wrinkles, mouth and eyelines and sagging cheeks by literally 'lifting' off part of the old face and replacing it.")

page 35: "topical or injected cocaine": see John B. Mulliken, M.D., "Biographical Sketch of Charles Conrad Miller, 'Featural Surgeon,' " *Plastic and Reconstructive Surgery,* February 1977, pp. 175–182. (According to Mulliken [p. 177], Miller, the first doctor in the U.S. to devote his practice to cosmetic surgery, "did his procedures in the office under local anesthesia, using a weak cocaine solution [one-quarter grain in one ounce of boiled water].")

page 35: " 'pioneer of the Peter Pan movement' ": Osbert Sitwell, "Charles and Charlemagne," *Dumb-Animal and Other Stories* (London: Duckworth, 1930), pp. 123, 154.

page 35: " 'They look like aliens' ": Amy Gross, "Very Plastic Surgery: What Are We Doing to Ourselves," *Elle,* March 1995, p. 50.

page 36: "people drink 'collagen cola' ": Dennis Dermody, "Cinemaniac: A Day in Celebrity Surgery Land," *Paper Guide,* Summer 1996, p. 128.

page 36: " 'Aging is difficult' ": Author's interview with Rees, June 1997.

page 36: "It took a cancer scare": Author's interview with Meg Cox, September 1996.

page 37: "an inspirational before-and-after story": Kathy Davis, *Reshaping the Female Body* (New York: Routledge, 1995), p. 167.

page 37: "her own face-lift": Diana McLellan, "Young Again!" *Washingtonian,* September 1989, pp. 160–172.

page 38: "may feel ashamed": Robert M. Goldwyn, M.D., *The Patient and the Plastic Surgeon* (Boston: Little, Brown and Company, 1991), p. 141.

page 40: "competitors to take similar measures": Joan Kron, "Nipping and Tucking in Tinseltown," *Allure*, May 1995, pp. 166–171.

page 40: "even an earthquake": Ibid.

page 41: "the invention of the close-up": Clive James, *Fame in the Twentieth Century* (New York: Random House, 1993), p. 30.

page 41: " 'We didn't need dialogue' ": quoted in Anthony Synnott, *The Body Social: Symbolism, Self and Society* (London: Routledge, 1993), p. 73.

page 41: "never lied about her age": Cornelia Otis Skinner, *Madame Sarah* (Boston: Houghton Mifflin Co., 1967), p. 328.

page 42: "regained a surprising degree of youthfulness": Madame Le Dr. A. Noël, *La Chirurgie Esthetique: Son Role Social* (Paris: Masson et Cie., 1926) pp. 5–6. (The English translation of the passages about the great actress can be found in Blair O. Rogers, M.D., "A Brief History of Cosmetic Surgery, *Surgical Clinics of North America* [Vol. 51, No. 2, April 1971], pp. 265–288. It was Bernhardt who inspired Dr. Noël to specialize in cosmetic surgery. Noël would eventually meet the star and operate on her.)

page 42: "greatest engineering feat": "Plastic Surgery for the Stage," *The New York Times*, August 16, 1923, p. 14, col. 4.

page 42: "deeply ambivalent about her own Jewishness": Marion Meade, *Dorothy Parker: What Fresh Hell Is This?* (New York: Penguin Books, 1989), p. 253.

page 42: " 'she had wanted to marry Eddie' ": Ibid., p. 40.

page 42: "Miss Brice boldly": "Plastic Surgery for the Stage," The *New York Times*, August 16, 1923, p. 14, col. 4.

page 42: "change their name from Kabotchnik": "Lets Kabotchniks Take Name of Cabot," *The New York Times*, August 15, 1923, p. 10, col. 3.

page 43: "the divorce papers": Barbara Grossman, *Funny Woman* (Bloomington, IL.: Indiana University Press, 1991), p. 168.

page 43: "Noses cost fifty dollars": Author's interview with Edward Lamont, M.D., September 1994.

page 43: "his older brother Albert": Elizabeth Haiken, *Venus Envy: A History of Cosmetic Surgery* (Baltimore: Johns Hopkins Press, 1997) p. 97.

page 43: "actor named Marlon Brando": Peter Manso, *Brando: The Biography* (New York: Hyperion, 1994), p. 105.

page 43: "Dietrich had her upper rear molars removed": Diane Ackerman, *A Natural History of Love* (New York: Random House, 1994), p. 188.

page 43: " 'conservatives may look askance' ": Geri Trotta, "The Business of Being Better Looking," *Look*, April 13, 1948, p. 79.

page 44: "getting nowhere fast": Patrick McGrady, Jr., *The Youth Doctors* (New York: Coward-McCann, 1968) pp. 193–194. (See also Donald Spoto, *Marilyn Monroe: The Biography* [New York: HarperPaperbacks, 1993], p. 181. There is no agreement on what procedures Monroe had or who performed them: In the author's 1995 interview with McGrady, he said he believed Dr. W. John Pangman operated on Monroe's chin. Spoto's book says Dr. Michael Gurdin operated on Monroe in 1949, removing "a slight bump of cartilage from the tip of Monroe's nose" and inserting a silicone impant in her jaw. In the author's 1995 interview with Dorothy Henderson, R.N.,—Gurdin's longtime nurse—Henderson said she recalls assisting at the operation and Pangman—a friend of Gurdin's—did the surgery in Gurdin's office, and only the chin was done, not the nose.)

page 44: " 'you should have cut your chin' ": Ibid.

page 44: " 'When my looks start to go' ": Jib Fowles, *Starstruck* (Washington, D.C.: Smithsonian Institution Press, 1992), p. 227.

page 45: "before Monroe's death": Author's interview with Rosemary Eckersley, October 1994.

page 45: "makeup tricks could take years off": author's interview with Helen Sandler (former movie-magazine editor and niece of film mogul Louis B. Mayer), October 1994. (During the filming of *A Guy Named Joe* (1943), says Sandler, "My uncle was upset that Irene Dunne"— who made $100,000 per film in 1940—"was so wrinkled they had to put gauze over the camera lens.")

page 45: "plaster cast of her head": Author's interview with Michael Westmore, October 1994. (With this stand-in, Westmore added, lighting technicians could spend hours—even days—getting the shadows just right.)

page 45: "male actors 'discovered facial folds' ": Joan Kron, "Nipping and Tucking in Tinseltown," *Allure*, May 1995, pp. 166–171.

page 46: "coming out party": Norma Lee Browning, *FaceLifts: Everything You Always Wanted to Know* (Garden City, NY: Doubleday & Company, 1982), pp. 206–207.

page 47: "seal of approval": Geri Trotta, "Cosmetic Plastic Surgery: An Up-To-Date Report," *Harpers Bazaar*, June 1960, pp. 101, 126.

page 47: "debunked several myths": Eugenia Harris, "Nine Myths About Face-Lifting," *McCall's*, June 1961, pp. 78–79, 182.

page 47: "If there was any doubt": Anonymous, "The Diary of a Face Lift," *Ladies Home Journal*, May 1962, pp. 28, 30, 32, 101.

page 47: " 'the most common of facial operations' ": "A Complete Chart of Plastic Surgery," *McCall's*, August 1964, pp. 56, 135.

page 47: "Diller underwent a face-lift": Phyllis Diller, "What Every Woman Should Know About My Face-lift," *Pageant*, June 1972, pp. 26–33.

page 48: "considered Diller his landmark": Author's interview with Rosemary Eckersley, Ashley's widow, October 1994.

page 48: "Because of Diller's forthrightness": Author's interview with A. Richard Grossman, M.D. (a former Ashley associate), October 1994.

page 49: "Jackie Gleason": "Up Front: What's Up Doc? Jackie Gleason Talks About His Four-and-a-Half-Hour Facelift," *People*, August 8, 1977, pp. 12–15. (Gleason, who was sixty-one years old, gave credit to his plastic surgeon, Miami's Ralph Millard.)

page 49: "Why not a little job under your chin?": Joan Rivers with Richard Meryman, *Still Talking* (New York: Turtle Bay Books/Random House, 1991), pp. 68–69. (Also, author's interview with Rivers, February 1993.)

page 49: "to emulate Roseanne": "My Lives," *The Independent* (London), April 30, 1994; *Toronto Sun*, April 19, 1994.

page 49: "Roseanne confessed she changed her nose": Andrew Wilson, "Who's Afraid of the Face in the Mirror?" *The Guardian* (London), June 20, 1994, p. T10.

page 49: "But moral positions can shift": Author's interview with Elvin Zook, M.D., former president of the American Society for Plastic and Reconstructive Surgery, February 1994. ("It is common for people to tell you cosmetic surgery is superfluous, until they want to look as good as they feel," says Zook. "Then they'll have it and often not admit it.")

page 49: " 'there's always that option' ": Suzy, "The Eye," *Women's Wear Daily*, November 9, 1994.

page 50: " 'destroys the star's intrinsic worth' ": Author's interview with Jib Fowles, August 1996.

page 50: " 'I had Zsa Zsa Gabor in my office' ": Author's interview with A. Richard Grossman, M.D., October 1994.

page 50: "a photographer behind every bush": author's interview with Edward Terino, M.D., April, 1998.

page 51: " 'an aesthetic thing' ": Suzy Menkes, *Windsor Style* (Topsfield, MA: Salem House Publishers, 1987), p. 147.

page 51: "slice-and-stitch description": Sally Bedell Smith, *Reflected Glory: The Life of Pamela Churchill Harriman* (New York: Simon & Schuster), 1996, p. 326.

page 51: "breast implants during filming": Julie Salamon, *The Devil's Candy: The Bonfire of the Vanities Goes to Hollywood* (New York: Delta, 1991), pp. 266–267.

page 51: " 'counterfeit twenty dollar bill' ": Jib Fowles, *Starstruck* (Washington, D.C.: Smithsonian Institution Press, 1992), p. 140.

page 51: "sacrifices herself for us": author's interview with Jib Fowles, August 27, 1996.

page 51: "wasn't *entirely* the result of her workouts": Valerie Kuklenski, "People: Fonda Uses Crawford," United Press International, November 19, 1995. ("Fonda admitted to having had cosmetic surgery on her face. 'Do I look pinched and pulled and peeled, like I'm trying to deny my age? No I don't,' she said defensively." Also, Associated Press, "Jane Sez Bod Was Cut Above Average," *New York Daily News,* May 24, 1995. "Jane Fonda says she went beyond the burn to sculpt her renowned body—she went for the scalpel. In June's *Fitness* magazine, Fonda admits that she had plastic surgery while married to Tom Hayden. But she wouldn't reveal which parts were nipped and tucked. 'I have had the basic amount of work done for people in the industry,' " said the actress.)

page 52: "more interested in the artifice": Joshua Gamson, *Claims to Fame: Celebrity in Contemporary America* (Berkeley: University of California Press, 1994), p. 147.

CHAPTER FOUR: FINDING DR. RIGHT

page 53: " 'Patients think beautiful hands are important' ": author's interview with Yves-Gérard Illouz, the French surgeon who developed liposuction, October 1995.

page 53: "There are more than 150 board-certified plastic surgeons in New York City": according to the 1997 roster of the American Society of Plastic and Reconstructive Surgeons.

page 54: "mutual selection process": author's interview with Brunno Ristow, M.D., October 1997.

page 56: "one West Coast surgeon asks his patients to take a psychological test." Author's interview with Edward Terino, M.D., February 1993.

page 56: "the choice of doctor is made 'more on the basis of trust than of knowledge' ": Robert M. Goldwyn, M.D. *The Patient and the Plastic Surgeon* (Boston: Little, Brown and Company, 1991), p. 48.

page 56: "Taste is the great match-maker": Pierre Bourdieu, *Distinction: A Social Critique of the Judgment of Taste* (Cambridge, MA: Harvard University Press, 1984), p. 241.

page 57: "Today anyone with an M.D. degree": 1997 position paper, American Society for Aesthetic Plastic Surgery, "What Everyone Should Know About Plastic Surgery Credentials."

page 58: " 'Any sensible woman knows' ": Norma Lee Browning, *Face-Lifts: Everything You Always Wanted to Know* (Garden City, NY: Doubleday & Company, 1981), pp. 192–193.

page 59: "Many reputable doctors refuse": Author's interview with Michael Kane, M.D., July 1996.

page 59: "Janine found her doctor through his advertisement on the Internet": Joan Kron, "Meeting Dr. Right," *Allure,* September 1997, pp. 128–136.

page 60: "when women are thinking of making an image change they head for the newsstand": "New Images: Just 'Do It'? No, Better Read Up a Bit First," *Adweek,* March 25, 1996.

page 60: " 'When I see on a patient's chart, "referred by a magazine' ": Joan Kron, "What Can Go Wrong," *Allure,* September 1996, pp. 242–249.

page 63: "There is no ABMS board with the word 'cosmetic' in its title": American Board of Medical Specialties fact sheet, December 1995.

page 64: "The medical board of California voted in July 1997 that doctors": Press Release, "Nationwide Protection Against Misleading Physician Advertisements: The California Model": Issued by the American Society for Aesthetic Plastic Surgery, undated (received by author December 17, 1997).

page 65: " 'nothing to stop anyone from incorporating' ": Author's interview with Michael Kane, M.D., July 1996.

page 65: " 'You have to learn what others have done' ': Frank McDowell. M.D., *The Source Book for Plastic Surgery* (Baltimore: Williams and Wilkins, 1977), p. vi.

page 66: "spawned a new field—the cosmetic-surgery matchmaker": Joan Kron, "Meeting Dr. Right," *Allure,* September 1997, pp. 128–136.

page 67: "According to laws in some states": Ibid.

page 69: "the doctors who would do such work 'charlatans' ": See Kathy Davis, *Reshaping the Female Body: The Dilemma of Cosmetic Surgery* (London: Routledge, 1995), p. 167. (Davis said there are five basic themes in magazine articles about plastic surgery: the "Before-and-After story"; "Success story"; "Celebrity story"; "Deviant story"; and "Atrocity story." Charlatans have long been staples of the "atrocity" genre.)

page 69: "as easy a mark for self-promoters as her grandmother": Mary Cable et al., *American Manners and Morals* (New York: American Heritage Publishing Co., 1969), pp. 258. ("Lydia Pinkham's Vegetable Compound, a best-selling herb syrup . . . was [promoted as] nature's remedy for the 'worst forms of Female Complaints.' ")

page 69: "a 'self-confessed [beauty surgery] faker' admitted": Anonymous, "The Truth About Beauty Surgery by an Ex-Plastic Surgeon," *Liberty,* January 17, 1925, pp. 5–7; *Liberty,* January 31, 1925, pp. 35–37; *Liberty,* February 14, 1925, pp. 34–35.

page 70: "The knave admitted to tricks of the trade": Ibid. (Considering that he took only one course in plastic surgery, the anonymous charlatan's range of treatments was awesome. He claimed to have given dimples to an actress who became known for them—the only problem, he said, was that "she had them even when she cried or frowned.")

page 70: "the original Doctor Wrong, Henry Junius Schireson": Morris Fishbein, M.D. "Twentieth-Century Charlatans," *Morris Fishbein, M.D., An Autobiography* (New York: Doubleday & Company, 1969), pp. 47–50.

page 70: "unethical for a reputable doctor": Pam Hait, "The History of the American Society of Plastic and Reconstructive Surgeons, Inc. 1931–1994" *Plastic and Reconstructive Surgery,* September 1994, p. 68A.

page 70: "so did the admonitions": Dorothy Cocks, "What About Plastic Surgery?" *Good Housekeeping,* June 1930, Volume 90, pp. 109, 150, 152. (In this article, a prominent doctor—unnamed—berates women for going to doctors on the recommendation of a "bridge teacher." The great doctor concluded that women's "secretiveness protects the 'charlatan' beauty surgeons." He apparently could not recognize the irony of keeping his own name a secret.)

page 71: " 'ratio to the skill of the surgeon' ": Lois Mattox Miller, "Surgery's Cinderella" *The Independent Woman,* July 1939, Volume 18, pp. 201, 222–223; Lois Mattox Miller, "Cinderella Surgery," *Reader's Digest,* August 1939, Vol. 35, pp. 84–86.

page 71: "Browning, 'a darling of the tabloids' ": Edward Lamont, M.D. "The Evolution of Aesthetic Plastic Surgery," Presented at the 17th annual meeting of the Japan Society of Aesthetic Plastic Surgery (Tokyo, Japan: October 18, 1994), pp. 21–22.

page 71: "that fat removal in the legs had been tried": J. Glicenstein, "L'Affaire Dujarier," *Annales Chirurgie Plastique Esthetique,* Vol. 34, No. 3, 1989, pp. 290–292.

page 71: "her face was 'smashed almost beyond recognition' ": David Grafton, *The Sisters: The Lives and Times of the Fabulous Cushing Sisters* (New York: Villard, 1992), p. 56.

page 71: " 'she didn't have her face reconstructed' ": Author's interview with Thomas D. Rees, M.D., October 1997.

page 71: "in 1937, the American Board of Plastic Surgery was formed": Pam Hait, "History of the American Society of Plastic and Reconstructive Surgeons," *Plastic and Reconstructive Surgery,* September 1994, Vol. 94., No. 4, p. 19A.

page 72: "put themselves in the hands of": Ruth Merrin, "A New Nose in a Week," *Good Housekeeping,* November 1940, Vol. III, pp. 82–83.

page 72: "reputable surgeons felt only the 'nasally desperate' deserved help": "Medicine: A Nose is a Nose is a Nose," *Time,* October 8, 1945, pp. 69–70.

page 72: "They became Weight Watchers in 1961": Lorraine Glennon, editor, *Our Times: Illustrated History of the Twentieth Century* (Atlanta: Turner Publishing, Inc., 1995), p. 456.

page 72: "touching off a major legal battle": Geri Trotta, "Cosmetic Plastic Surgery: Up-to-Date Report," *Harper's Bazaar,* June 1960, pp. 101, 126.

page 72: "E.N.T. specialists were 'outraged' ": "History of the American Society of Plastic and Reconstructive Surgeons, Inc. 1931–1994.", pp. 56A–59A, 73A.

page 72: "when she showed her staff graphic, under-the-skin pictures": Diana Vreeland with Christopher Hemphill, *Allure* (Garden City, NY: Doubleday, 1980), pp. 136–137.

page 73: "The breakthrough article": Simona Morini, "Body Sculpting: New Techniques in Cosmetic Surgery for Every Part of the Body . . . and a Working Day in the Life of an Internationally Famous Doctor," *Vogue*, October 1, 1969, pp. 190–194, 259.

page 73: " 'the roof fell off the building!' ": Mark Hampton and Mary Louise Wilson, *Full Gallop* (Dramatists Play Service, 1996), pp. 34–35. Excerpted with permission. (In the one-woman show, based on Vreeland's memoirs, Vreeland revels in having been the first editor to demystify cosmetic surgery and in the brouhaha the subject caused with *Vogue*'s management. "We had an awful battle over the piece I published on plastic surgery . . . Of course," she says with typical exaggeration, "people have been having face-lifts since the time of the Romans.")

page 73: "Rio taxi drivers knew": Simona Morini, "Body Sculpting: New Techniques in Cosmetic Surgery for Every Part of the Body . . . and a Working Day in the Life of an Internationally Famous Doctor," *Vogue*, October 1, 1969, pp. 190–194, 259.

page 73: "Even today, on Park Avenue": Joan Kron, "The Nip-and-Tuck Career of Ivo Pitanguy," *Allure*, September 1994, pp. 194–199, 230–231.

page 73: " 'The consequences [of self-promotion] were severe' ": Author's interview with Thomas D. Rees, M.D. July 1994.

page 74: " 'If I didn't think this had value' ": Author's interview with Ivo Pitanguy, M.D., November 1996.

page 75: " 'Man has always sought to be similar' ": Ivo Pitanguy, M.D., "Creativity and Plastic Surgery," *Revista Brasileira de Cirurgia*, Vol. 83, No. 2, 1993, pp. 79–86.

page 75: " 'It was a slice of high life' ": Author's interview with Eleanor Lambert, June 1994.

page 75: " 'they would have lost their licenses' ": Joan Kron, "The Nip and Tuck Career of Ivo Pitanguy," *Allure*, September 1994, pp. 194–199, 230–231.

page 76: "The photo of 'Doctor Vanity' ": Warren Hoge, "Doctor Vanity: The Jet Set's Man in Rio," *The New York Times Magazine*, June 8, 1980, pp. 42–46, 52–68.

page 76: " 'Not everyone ages equally well' ": Author's interview with Ivo Pitanguy, M.D., October 1996.

page 76: "there is no correlation between level of a cosmetic surgeon's skill": Daniel Kagan, "The Hard Facts About Cosmetic Surgery," *Mademoiselle*, November 1986, pp. 248–249.

page 76: "coined the term 'scalpel slaves' ": Jennet Conant et al., "Scalpel Slaves Just Can't Quit," *Newsweek*, January 11, 1988, p. 58.

page 76: "the phenomenon of the surgical redo": Susan Jacoby, "The Cosmetic Surgery Boom," *Glamour*, March 1988, pp. 292–293, 348–352.

page 77: "advertising had given plastic surgery": Jerry Adler et al. "New Bodies for Sale," *Newsweek*, May 27, 1985, p. 64.

page 77: "investigated by New York State": Ibid.

page 77: "lost his medical license": Laura Muha, "Court OKs Paying Victims of 'Personal Best' Surgeon,": *Newsday*, September 20, 1990, p. 6; Adam Z. Horvath, "Victims Who Wait: Cash Slow to Reach Convicted MD's Patients," *Newsday*, January 2, 1990, p. 2.

page 77: "a totally unfounded rumor": Thomas D. Rees, M.D., "A Rumor of AIDS," *New York*, August 2, 1993, pp. 26–32.

CHAPTER FIVE: LIFE AND DEATH DETAILS

page 81: " 'God is in the details.' ": Ludwig Mies van der Rohe and Gustave Flaubert (unverified), *Bartlett's Familiar Quotations* (Boston: Little, Brown & Co., 1998).

page 82: "to illustrate the hideous disfigurements": Blair O. Rogers, M.D., "The First Pre- and Post-Operative Photographs of Plastic and Reconstructive Surgery: Contributions of Gurdon Buck (1807–1877)," *Aesthetic Plastic Surgery*, No. 15, 1991, pp. 19–33.

page 84: "Jewelry and makeup are considered": Harvey A. Zarem, "Standards of Photography," *Plastic and Reconstructive Surgery*, July 1984, pp. 137–146.

page 85: "Attractiveness is fleeting": Robin Tolmach Lakoff and Raquel L. Scherr, *Face Value: The Politics of Beauty* (Boston: Routledge & Kegan Paul, 1984), pp. 19–20.

page 86: " 'she smashed a statue of herself' ": Sharon Romm, M.D., *The Changing Face of Beauty* (St. Louis: Mosby Year Book, 1992), p. 74.

page 90: "being kept warm is crucial": "Health Report," *Time*, April 21, 1997, p. 36.

page 90: "blood clots better": Author's interview with Tom Nyberg, M.D., January 1998.

page 92: "taking the anti-depresant": remarks of dermatologist Rhoda Narins at an annual meeting of the American Society of Dermatological Surgery, Boston, May 1997.

page 92: "stop supplements of vitamin E": Jane E. Brody, "In Vitamin Mania, Millions Take a Gamble on Health," *The New York Times*, October 26, 1997, pp. 1, 28, 29. (Brody explains that high doses of vitamin E "interfere with absorption of . . . vitamin K, which promotes blood clotting: supplements should not be taken before surgery.")

page 96: "statistics improve every year": Author's interview with E. S. Siker, M.D., May 1996 (Siker is the founder of the Anesthesia Patient Safety Association.) Statistics are from American Society of Anesthesiologists, Park Ridge, IL.

page 97: "allergic reaction to anesthesia": Author's interview with anesthesiologist L. David Silver, M.D., April 1996 ("In fifteen years of practice," says Silver, "I have never seen an allergic reaction to anesthesia.")

page 100: "elevated blood pressure before an operation": Author's interview with Alan Matarasso, M.D., May 1996. (In a study conducted by Matarasso of blepharoplasty done under purely local anesthesia, 25 percent of patients had a dangerous change of heart rate, which may be related to anxiety. He advises cardiac monitoring even with local anesthesia.)

page 100: "Most face-lifts were done under local": John Q. Owsley, M.D., *Aesthetic Facial Surgery* (Philadelphia: W. B. Saunders, 1994), p. 38. ("For many years, I used local anesthesia," Owsley writes, "but as the operation became more technically complex and lengthy and often combined with multiple associated procedures, I turned to general anesthesia.")

page 103: "history of severe nausea after general anesthesia": John Bornstein, M.D., Martin Gordon, M.D., and Steven M. Hoefflin, M.D., "A Sixteen Year Experience With a Personalized Plastic Surgery General Anesthesia Program: A Report on Over 20,000 Procedures Without Any Significant Complications," 1997, unpublished.

CHAPTER SIX: ANATOMY OF A FACE-LIFT

page 105: "It is not everybody's good fortune": Anthony F. Wallace, *The Progress of Plastic Surgery: An Introductory History* (Oxford, England: Willem A. Meeuws, 1982), pp. 105–106.

page 105: "a little work on her jawline": Liz Smith, "Frank's Day in May," *Newsday*, January 9, 1998, p. A15.

page 106: "he once amputated a leg": Blair O. Rogers, M.D., "A Chronological History of Cosmetic Surgery," *Bulletin of the New York Academy of Medicine, Second Series*, Vol. 47, No. 3, March 1971, pp. 265–302.

page 107: "he blamed 'feminine persuasion' ": Ibid.

page 108: " 'Even the Brothers Mayo would have flinched' ": S. J. Perelman, "Mid-Winter Trends, *The Best of S. J. Perelman* (New York: Random House, 1947), pp. 113–117.

page 108: "a most profitable and satisfactory specialty": Blair O. Rogers, M.D., "A Chronological History of Cosmetic Surgery," *Bulletin of the New York Academy of Medicine, Second Series*, Vol. 47, No. 3, March 1971, pp. 265–302. (Miller churned out a prodigious number of papers describing his techniques. His 1907 book, *Cosmetic Surgery: The Correction of Featural Imperfections*, is considered the first textbook on the cosmetic surgery. According to Rogers, Miller was both a "quack" and a "visionary." He was the first to describe how to create dimples. For wrinkles he promoted injections of paraffin, which proved to be disastrous. He experimented with other questionable fillers such as silk, celluloid, vegetable ivory, sponge rubber, and gutta percha, which he pulverized in a spinach grinder. They all proved to be dangerous or useless.)

page 108: "had her nose 'tip-tilted' ": Felicia Warburg Roosevelt, *Doers and Dowagers* (Garden City, New York: Doubleday & Company, 1975), pp. 216–217.

page 108: "needed to look younger": See Blair O. Rogers, M.D., "A Chronological History of Cosmetic Surgery," *Bulletin of the New York Academy of Medicine, Second Series,* Vol. 47, No. 3, March 1971, pp. 265–302 for examples.

page 108: "There was an adage in the U.S.": Mary Cable et al., *American Manners & Morals,* (New York: American Heritage Publishing, 1969), p. 295.

page 108: "she intended to marry a man": Blair O. Rogers, M.D., "A Chronological History of Plastic Surgery," *Bulletin of the New York Academy of Medicine, Second Series,* Vol. 47, No. 3, March 1971, pp. 265–302.

page 109: "a 1926 British book promised": Charles H. Willi, *Facial Rejuvenation: How to Idealize the Features and the Skin of the Face by Latest Scientific Methods* (London: Cecil Palmer, 1926), p. x.

page 109: "Bernhardt who inspired Noël's interest": Mme. Le Dr A. Noël, *La Chirurgie Esthetique: Son Role Social* (Paris: Masson et Cie., 1926), p. 5. (According to Cornelia Otis Skinner, in *Madame Sarah* [Boston: Houghton Mifflin Company, 1967], pp. 306–313, Bernhardt toured the U.S. in 1910–11.

page 109: "Bernhardt was the actress": Author's interview with Paule Regnault, F.R.C.S., September 1995; and author's interview with Claude Perpere, M.D., November 1995.

page 110: "her landmark 1926 textbook": Mme. Le Dr A. Noël, *La Chirurgie Esthetique: Son Role Social* (Paris: Masson et Cie., 1926).

page 110: "not wearing gloves": Ibid. (See also Paule Regnault, F.R.C.S. and Kathryn Stephenson, M.D., "Dr. Suzanne Noël: The First Woman to do Esthetic Surgery," *Plastic and Reconstructive Surgery,* August 1971, Vol. 48, No. 2., pp. 133–139. Regnault worked with Noël from 1942 to 1950, earning one dollar for assisting with a face-lift and two dollars for a breast reduction. Regnault recalls Noël operating once wearing a watch but no surgical gloves. "Don't worry," Noël told her, "this watch is very good.")

page 110: "dressed in an evening gown": Judith B. Zacher, "Plastic Surgery in the Late 1920s," *Clinics in Plastic Surgery: Historical Perspectives of Plastic Surgery* (Philadelphia: W. B. Saunders Company), October 1983, Vol. 10, No. 4, pp. 665–667.

page 111: "a recent European study": Conducted by Vladimir Mitz, M.D. and Yaron Yarshai, M.D.

page 111: "once you see the result": Author's interview with Sherrell J. Aston, M.D., January 1998.

page 111: "just pull the skin up and back": Joan Kron, "Dueling Face-Lifts," *Allure*, August 1996, pp. 82, 84, 86, 99.

page 112: "Rees's ideal patient": Thomas D. Rees, M.D. and Donald Wood-Smith, M.D. *Cosmetic Facial Surgery* (Philadelphia: W. B. Saunders Company, 1973), p. 136.

page 112: "key to a longer-lasting lift": Tord Skoog, *Plastic Surgery: New Methods and Refinements,* (Philadelphia: W. B. Saunders, 1974).

page 113: " 'The Skoog woman' ": Author's interview with John N. Yousif, M.D., November 1997.

page 113: " 'May be helpful in face-lift operations' ": Vladimir Mitz and Martine Peyronie, "The Superficial Musculo-Aponeurotic System (SMAS) in the Parotid and Cheek Area," *Plastic and Reconstructive Surgery*, Vol. 58, No. 80, 1976.

page 113: " 'Good for seven to ten years' ": Melva Weber, "Plastic Update: Ways to Keep the Look of Youth," *Vogue*, October 1983, pp. 385, 388.

page 115: "incrementally, as early as needed": Gerald Imber, M.D., *The Youth Corridor* (New York: William Morrow Company, 1997), p. xii. (Imber believes in "preventing wrinkles, rather than curing them, and smaller procedures and earlier surgery for generally younger patients.")

page 115: " 'Do it all at once' ": Joan Kron, "Dueling Face-Lifts," *Allure*, August 1996, pp. 82, 84, 86, 99. Hamra's technique is described in detail in Sam T. Hamra, M.D., "Composite Rhytidectomy," (St. Louis: Quality Medical Publishing, 1993).

page 116: "neck anatomy varies": See Sherrell, J. Aston, M.D., "Platysma Muscle in Rhytidoplasty," *Annals of Plastic Surgery*, 1979, 3:6.

page 116: "It took a world-famous beauty": Author's interview with Docteur Yves-Gérard Illouz, New York, October 1995.

page 117: "can't be pulled tight enough": Author's interview with Joseph G. McCarthy, M.D., November 1997.

page 117: " 'Don't make it too tight' ": Joel Feldman, M.D.'s, comments during his teaching course on aesthetic neck surgery, at American Society of Plastic and Reconstructive Surgeons conference in San Francisco, November 1997.

page 120: " 'noses don't grow' ": Author's interview with Jack P. Gunter, M.D., October 1996.

page 121: "took a swipe at Jennifer": "Page Six," *New York Post*, October 29, 1997.

page 121: "I submitted my face": Author's interview with Gilbert Aiach, M.D., June 1993.

page 122: "post-modern 'metamorph' ": Joan Kron, "Body Makeover," *Allure*, March 1993, pp. 136–139, 164. (Metamorph is a word coined by McCracken in conversation with author.)

page 122: "hooked nose a symbol of power": John Conley, M.D., *Face-Lift Operation* (Springfield, Illinois: Charles C. Thomas, Publisher, 1968), p. 7.

page 123: " 'want a new nose, pay me a visit' ": Solomon R. Kagan, M.D., *Jewish Contributions to Medicine in America from Colonial Times to the Present* (Boston: Boston Medical Publishing Co., 1939), p. 4.

page 123: "it was called the 'Italian operation' ": Martha Teach Gnudi and Jerome Pierce Webster, *The Life and Times of Gaspare Tagliacozzi, Surgeon of Bologna 1545–1599* (New York: Herbert Reichner, 1950). Tagliacozzi's landmark book, *De curtorum Chirurgia per insitionem* (Venice: 1597) was the first volume devoted to plastic surgery.

page 123: "mecca for European nobles": Solomon R. Kagan, M.D., *Jewish Contributions to Medicine in America from Colonial Times to the Present* (Boston: Boston Medical Publishing Co., 1939), p. 5. (At one time, wrote Kagan, Tagliacozzi "had under his care twelve German counts, nineteen French marquises, and one hundred Spanish cavaliers, besides one solitary English esquire.")

page 124: "the ideal nose was 'well-made' ": Richard Corson, *Fashions in Makeup* (New York: Universe Books, 1972), p. 172.

page 124: "If anesthesia had been around": Helen Bransford, *Welcome to Your Facelift* (Garden City, New York: Doubleday, 1997), p. 39.

page 124: "The Egyptians used mandrake": Lise Manniche, *An Ancient Egyptian Herbal*, (Austin, Texas: University of Texas Press, 1989); Sherwin B. Nuland, "Surgery Without Pain: The Origins of General Anesthesia," *Doctors: A Biography of Medicine*, (New York: Vintage Books, 1995) pp. 263–303. (According to Nuland, the Greeks' "narke"—narcotic—was opium, derived from the sap of the poppy. Dioscorides, the chief surgeon of Nero's Roman army and an authority on herbal medicine, induced sleep with the plant henbane. Pliny, the Elder, a Roman naturalist, recommended the juice of the mandragora—mandrake—"before the cutting, cauterizing, pricking, or lancing of any member, to take away the sense and feeling." These herbs were still in use in the Middle Ages, when cocktails of opium, mulberry juice, lettuce seed, hemlock, mandrake, ivy, and Hyoscyamus were employed. Fennel juice or vinegar was the post-op waker-upper. There wasn't much incentive to find anything better, wrote Nuland, because pain, according to the Christian theological doctrine, "served God's purpose." In the nineteenth century, mesmerism, a form of hypnosis, and later nitrous oxide and ether, introduced as novelties at ether frolics and laughing-gas parties, proved effective for surgery. William Morton, who discovered ether, called it Letheon, the same name popularized by Virgil to "refer to poppy-induced sleep.")

page 124: "what Cleopatra VII looked like": Lucy Hughes-Hallett, *Cleopatra: Histories, Dreams and Distortions* (New York: Harper & Row Publishers, 1990), pp. 17, 63, 67–68, 137, 179, 220, 256.

page 125: "descriptions written after her death are conflicting": Author's communication with Marsha Hill, Department of Egyptian Art, The Metropolitan Museum of Art, June

1997; Robert S. Bianchi et al., *Cleopatra's Egypt: Age of the Ptolemies* (New York: The Brooklyn Museum, 1988), pp. 159–164, 184–188. (Catalogue of a traveling exhibition organized by the Brooklyn Museum. Pictured here are the coins with Cleopatra's portraits.) See also Margaret George, "Author's Note," *The Memoirs of Cleopatra, a Novel* (New York: St. Martin's Press, 1997), pp. 958–963.

page 125: "If Cleopatra had wanted a nose job": Author's communication with Jacque Lynn Foltyn, Ph.D., June 1997.

page 126: "the ideal was of 'moderate size' ": Richard Corson, *Fashions in Makeup From Ancient to Modern Times*, (New York: Universe Books, 1972), p. 228.

page 126: " 'physiognomic reasoning' ": Grace Rees, *Character Reading from the Face: The Science of Physiognomy* (Kingswood, Surrey: Andrew George Elliot, 1950), pp. 42–43. (Quoted in Corrigan, Peter. *The Sociology of Consumption* [London: Sage Publications, 1997], pp. 158–159.)

page 126: "quills through my nostrils": John Conley, M.D., *Face-Lift Operation* (Springfield, Illinois: Charles C. Thomas, 1968), p. 6.

page 127: "typical middle-age female nose patient": James W. Fox, IV, M.D., "Aesthetic Rhinoplasty," in Robert William Bernard,, M.D., *Surgical Restoration of the Aging Face*, (Boston: Butterworth-Heinemann, 1996), pp. 229–248.

page 127: "even children with birth defects": Author's interview with Joseph G. McCarthy, M.D., director of the Institute of Reconstructive Plastic Surgery, New York University, April 1997.

page 127: " 'I offered to put the hump back' ": Author's interview with Jack Sheen, M.D., October 1995.

page 127: "four surgeons have been murdered by them": Joan Kron, "Appointment with Death," *Allure*, February 1994, pp. 102–105, 147. ("The Male Risk Factor," p. 105.)

page 127: "he previewed the effects": Peter Whitmer Ph.D., *The Inner Elvis: A Psychological Biography of Elvis Aaron Presley* (New York: Hyperion, 1960). (Described in John O'Mahony, "Elvis Used Pals as Surgery Guinea Pigs," *New York Post*, August 11, 1996, p. 34.)

page 128: "he might have known that two Americans": Frank McDowell, M.D., *The Source Book for Plastic Surgery* (Baltimore: Williams and Wilkins, 1977), p. 114–120.

page 128: "the rich and royal": Paul Natvig, *Jacques Joseph: Surgical Sculptor* (Philadelphia: W. B. Saunders Company, 1982), page 50.

page 129: "four psychological types": Prof. Dr. J. Joseph, *Rhinoplasty and Facial Plastic Surgery* (Phoenix: Columella Press, 1987) pp. 36–39.

page 129: "Some say Joseph put a gun in his mouth": Frank McDowell. M.D., *The Source Book for Plastic Surgery* (Baltimore: Williams and Wilkins, 1977), p. 177. (According to McDowell, "there is a good bit of uncertainty about the manner of Joseph's death.")

page 130: "estrogen can loosen": author's interview with Robert Flowers, M.D., November 1997.

page 130: "the number-one facial procedure": There were 159,232 blepharoplasties performed in 1997 according to "ASAPS 1997 Statistics on Cosmetic Surgery" (New York: American Society for Aesthetic Plastic Surgery, 1998).

page 132: "four cases of punctured eyeballs reported": Thomas L. Roberts, III, M.D., "Overview of Applications of CO2 Lasers"; and Richard Gregory, M.D., "Comparisons of CO2 Lasers," presentations at "Advances in Aesthetic Plastic Surgery: The Cutting Edge," a meeting sponsored by Manhattan Eye Ear & Throat Hospital, October 1–5, 1996; also, author's interviews with Norman Shorr, M.D., and Richard Lisman, M.D., March 1998.

page 132: "they clamped the excess skin": Anthony F. Wallace, *The Progress of Plastic Surgery: An Introductory History* (Oxford, England: William A. Meeuws, 1982), pp. 100, 101.

page 136: "6 to 16 percent in African populations": Press release, BioSpecifics Technologies Corp, "Promising Early Results for Keloid Treatment Reported at 1997 Conference on the International Burn Foundation," February 25, 1997.

page 136: "keloid scar on eyelid": Author's interview with Sherrell J. Aston, M.D., January 1998.

page 137: "the post-tragal incision": Thomas D. Rees, "In Search of the Perfect Face-Lift: A Personal Odyssey." *Aesthetic Surgery,* January/February 1997, pp. 29–36.

CHAPTER SEVEN: PRESSING OUT THE WRINKLES

page 139: " 'It's not the age' ": *Raiders of the Lost Ark,* 1981.

page 142: "accenting their natural wrinkle lines with makeup": Serge Strenkovsky, *The Art of Makeup* (New York: E. P. Dutton, 1943), p. 199.

page 143: " 'the furrows that signify how we have pondered' ": Mary Tannen, "Why the Knife?" *Allure,* October 1992, pp. 88–90.

page 143: "ghosts of the myriad": Charles Seibert, "Effacing Ourselves," *The New York Times Magazine,* July 7, 1996, pp. 20–25, 34, 40, 43–45.

page 143: "an obscure fruit called the 'hemayet' ": Lise Manniche, *An Ancient Herbal* (Austin: University of Texas Press, 1989), pp. 151–152. (This is sometimes spelled hmæyt.)

page 143: "hype in a bottle": James Henry Breasted, *The Edwin Smith Surgical Papyrus* (Chicago: University of Chicago Press, 1930, vol. 1), pp. 506–507. Also see Willard L. Marmelzat, M.D., "Bits of History, Bits of Mystery: A Historical Review of Chemical Rejuvenation of the Face," in Robert Kotler, M.D., *Chemical Rejuvenation of the Face* (St. Louis: Mosby Year Book, 1992), p. 3.

page 144: "oatmeal paste and lemon juice": Lillian Eichler, *The Customs of Mankind* (Doubleday, Page & Company, 1924), p. 558.

page 144: "beauty masks of clay": Ibid, p. 556.

page 144: "ointments made with 'narcissus bulbs' ": Sharon Romm, M.D., *The Changing Face of Beauty* (St. Louis: Mosby Year Book, 1992), p. 205.

page 144: " 'turn Hecuba into Helen' ": Willard L. Marmelzat, M.D., "Bits of History, Bits of Mystery: A Historical Review of Chemical Rejuvenation of the Face," in Robert Kotler, M.D., *Chemical Rejuvenation of the Face* (St. Louis: Mosby Year Book, 1992), p. 5.

page 144: "Elizabeth I smoothed her forehead creases": Sharon Romm, M.D., *The Changing Face of Beauty* (St. Louis: Mosby Year Book, 1992), pp. 208–211.

page 145: " 'cosmetology did not belong in medicine.' ": Willard L. Marmelzat, M.D., "Bits of History, Bits of Mystery: A Historical Review of Chemical Rejuvenation of the Face," in Robert Kotler, M.D., *Chemical Rejuvenation of the Face* (St. Louis: Mosby Year Book, 1992), p. 8.

page 145: "ingest chalk, poisonous arsenic": Lois W. Banner, *American Beauty* (Chicago: University of Chicago Press, 1983), pp. 40–14.

page 145: " 'skinning' (or *encorchement* . . .)": Lois W. Banner, *American Beauty* (Chicago: University of Chicago Press, 1983), pp. 213–215.

page 145: "skinning had left one girl's face": Elizabeth Boyd, "My Experiences in Wanting to Be Beautiful," *Ladies Home Journal*, January 1908, pp. 17–18.

page 146: "phenol is alive and well": Author's interview with Phillip A. Stone, M.D., January 1998; see also Phillip A. Stone, M.D., "The Use of Modified Phenol for Chemical Face Peeling," *Clinics in Plastic Surgery: Skin Resurfacing* (Philadelphia: W. B. Saunders, January 1998), pp. 21–44.

page 148: "Mae West, who was forty in 1932": James Monaco et al., *The Encyclopedia of Film* (New York: Perigee/Putnam, 1991), p. 573.

page 148: "developed a droopy eyelid": Author's interview with Richard Aronsohn, M.D., November 1994.

page 148: "soon eclipsed by Jean De Desley": Author's interview with Arthur Gradé, October 1994. (Gradé believed that De Desley was the former silent film actress Jean Ferguson, but I cannot verify that. Her death certificate shows she was born in Mississippi on November 20, 1891, née Maime Elizabeth Larson, was married to Norman Disley of Panorama City, California, and died on February 3, 1973.)

page 148: "many believed she was the legendary 'Lady in Black' ": See Valentino biography in Lorraine Glennon, ed., *Our Times: The Illustrated History of the Twentieth Century* (Atlanta: Turner Publishing, 1995), p. 162.

page 148: "One of De Desley's students . . . was Sarah Shaw": Hurley R. Taplis, "To Whom it May Concern" (facsimile of notorized letter), dated October 15, 1953. Taplis, a Los Angeles lawyer, was one of the attorneys of record in the Will Contest in the Estate of Antoinette La Gassé. The letter states that "Mrs. Desley testified under oath that in . . . approximately . . . 1926, she taught Antoinette La Gassé, who was then known as Sarah Shaw, all of the techniques, arts, and skills later used by Miss La Gassé in facial rejuvenation, beauty treatments, etc. . . . Her testimony was not disputed." From "documentary evidence . . . signed by Miss La Gassé, the proof is conclusive," stated Talpis, "that Mrs. Desley taught Antoinette La Gassé." (Letter sent to author by Arthur Gradé, October 1994.)

page 148: "turns up as medical fact": Thomas J. Baker, M.D., James M. Stuzin, M.D., and Tracy M. Baker, M.D., *Facial Skin Resurfacing* (St. Louis: Quality Medical Publishing, Inc., 1998), p. 4.

page 149: "putting anything stronger . . . on someone's face is and was a felony": If the peeling agent induces a physiological change in living cells (as phenol and medium strength trichloroacetic acid does), then it is considered a medical treatment and the agent is considered a drug and must be administered by a physician. If it is an agent like glycolic acid (a fruit acid) that removes the dead cell layer of skin (the keratin layer), then the agent can be administered by office personnel or an esthetician.

page 149: "Fountain of Youth Ranch": Ruthe Deskin, "Untitled" (pre-publication galley of Cora Galenti obituary), *Las Vegas Sun*, dated September 9, 1993 (presumably for the September 10 edition); author's interview with Ruthe Deskin, October 1994.

page 149: "the treatment felt 'like liquid fire' ": Patrick McGrady, Jr., *The Youth Doctors* (New York: Coward-McCann, Inc., 1968), pp. 221–250.

page 151: "sheep-cell therapy": Ibid, pp. 79–85, 130.

page 151: "painting on the acid": Author's interview with Edward J. Truppman, M.D., March 1995.

page 151: "It was like painting the White House": Author's interview with Edward J. Truppman, M.D., March 1995.

page 151: "Ointments and compresses were applied on subsequent days": Author's interview with Richard Aronsohn, M.D., November 1994.

page 151: "thank-you note . . . on flowered stationery": Facsimile, Lana Turner's letter to Arthur Gradé, March 25, 1977 (received by author from Arthur Gradé, October 15, 1994), 2 pages.

page 151: " 'the Tiffany of lady face-peelers.' ": Clipping in Venner Kelsen's scrapbooks, marked "What Helen Gould of *Coronet Magazine* (July 1970) says about Venner Kelsen and her remarkable facial rejuvenation"; author's interview with Vera Brown (the Kelsen protégé who inherited her effects), October 1994.

page 152: " 'women in Beverly Hills looked like ghosts' ": Author's interview with Jacque Thomas. (Thomas says Kelsen "made me swear I would never reveal the formulas and for a long while, I didn't. But now I believe it's not the formula that's so unique. The real secret was her technique—and the Rejuv Tape by Zauder Brothers, a New York costume company. They are out of business. I still have some—I bought a case. I don't know what I'll do when it runs out. Venner said the tape sculpts the face. The tape is removed at the end of the peel. Most doctors anesthetize the patient to take the tape off. We just lifted it off. It wasn't that painful. I have a picture of three of her New York ladies—in a penthouse—playing cards with tape on their faces.")

page 153: "the House of Renaissance": Jane and Michael Stern, *Encyclopedia of Bad Taste* (New York: Harper Collins, 1990), p. 112; Author's interview with Edward J. Truppman, M.D., March 1995.

page 153: "the Mascheks received national attention": Norma Lee Browning, *Face-Lifts: Everything You Always Wanted to Know* (Garden City, New York: Doubleday & Company, Inc., 1982), p. 68; also Author's interview with Browning, February 1997. (According to Browning, the series ran in 1960.)

page 153: "believing the series was a 'hoax.' ": Thomas J. Baker, M.D. and Howard L. Gordon, M.D., *Surgical Rejuvenation of the Face* (St. Louis: The C.V. Mosby Co., 1986), p. 44.

page 153: "on his own freckled forearm.": Thomas J. Baker, M.D., James M. Stuzin, M.D., and Tracy M. Baker, M.D., *Facial Skin Resurfacing* (St. Louis: Quality Medical Publishing, Inc., 1998), p. 45.

page 153: " 'It took a lot of courage' ": Willard L. Marmelzat, M.D., "Bits of History, Bits of Mystery: A Historical Review of Chemical Rejuvenation of the Face," in Robert Kotler, M.D., *Chemical Rejuvenation of the Face* (St. Louis: Mosby Year Book, 1992), p. 42.

page 154: "had a colorful and controversial career": Author's interview with Jacqueline Stallone, October 1994; Suzanne Adelson et al., "License to Kill?" *People,* July 26, 1982, p. 20.

page 154: "a Nevada plastic surgeon": Presentation by Gregory Hetter, M.D. at the meeting of the American Society for Aesthetic Plastic Surgery, New York, May 1997.

page 154: "sandpaper spinning at 10,000 revolutions": Willard L. Marmelzat, M.D., "Bits of History, Bits of Mystery: A Historical Review of Chemical Rejuvenation of the Face," in Robert Kotler, M.D., *Chemical Rejuvenation of the Face* (St. Louis: Mosby Year Book, 1992), p. 29.

page 155: "skin aging, 'is a chronic disease' ": Mark G. Rubin, M.D., *Manual of Chemical Peels* (Philadelphia: J. B. Lippincott, 1995), p. vii.

page 156: "I wrote an article about it": Joan Kron, "Friendly Fire," *Allure,* June 1995, pp. 100, 102, 104, 119.

page 157: "the first talk-show host to have his crows' feet zapped": Geraldo's laser doctor was Alan Gaynor, M.D.

page 158: "feeling 'like a Neanderthal.' ": Author's interview with Daniel Weiner, M.D., March 1997.

page 158: "cases of eyeball perforation": Author's interviews with Richard Lisman, M.D. and Norman Shorr, M.D., March 1998.

page 159: "followed a woman through a full-face laser peel": Sylvia Chase, *Prime Time Live*, May 1996.

page 160: "8 to 12 percent of patients": David B. Apfelberg, M.D., "Side Effects, Sequelae, and Complications of Carbon Dioxide Laser Resurfacing," *Aesthetic Surgery Journal*, November/December 1997, pp. 365–372.

page 162: "not approved by the FDA": "Physicians to Stop Injecting Silicone for Cosmetic Treatment of Wrinkles," Food and Drug Administration Press Release, February 28, 1992.

page 162: "form nodules of tissue.": "Liquid Injectable Silicone: Revised Position Paper," American Society for Aesthetic Plastic Surgery, December 1994.

page 162: "putting Plexiglas in my face": Gottfried Lemperle, M.D., Nelly Hazan-Gauthier, M.D., and Martin Lemperle, M.D., "PMMA Microspheres (Artecoll) for Skin and Soft-Tissue Augmentation. Part II: Clinical Investigations," *Plastic and Reconstructive Surgery*, September 1995, pp. 627–634.

page 163: "Even Andy Warhol confessed": Kennedy Fraser, *Scenes from the Fashionable World* (New York: Knopf, 1997), p. 197.

page 164: "the girl who wanted 'Sunken Cheeks Made Plump' ": "When Women Go to 'Beauty Parlors,' " *Ladies Home Journal*, November 1912, p. 14.

page 164: "Solid grease wasn't any better": Charles H. Willi, *Facial Rejuvenation: How to Idealize the Features and the Skin of the Face by the Latest Scientific Methods* (London: Cecil Palmer, 1926), p. 92.

page 164: "She became a recluse": Robert M. Goldwyn, M.D. "The Paraffin Story," *Plastic and Reconstructive Surgery*, April 1980, pp. 517–524.

page 164: "Liquid silicone was touted as": Pam Hait, "History of the American Society of Plastic and Reconstructive Surgeons, Inc., 1931–1994," *Plastic and Reconstructive Surgery*, September 1994, Vol. 94, No. 4, p. 59A.

page 164: " 'a sensational discovery' with great promise": Simona Morini, "A New Aid to Plastic Surgery: Silicone," *Vogue*, March 15, 1971, pp. 84–87, 114, 115.

page 165: "Jolie Gabor, mother of Zsa Zsa": Jolie Gabor and Cindy Adams, *Jolie Gabor as told to Cindy Adams* (New York: Mason Charter, 1975), pp. 298–299.

page 166: "Eileen Ford, owner of Ford Models": Ken Siman, *The Beauty Trip* (Pocket Books, 1995), p. 45.

page 166: "One of the most visible and outspoken casualties": Ann Louise Bardach, "The Dark Side of Plastic Surgery," *The New York Times*, April 17, 1988, Section 6, part 2, p. 24, column 1. (Young's doctor, Jack Starz—who later killed himself—had, according to *The Times*, 105 other lawsuits.)

page 166: "she has given interviews": Ann Louise Bardach, "The Dark Side of Plastic Surgery," *The New York Times*, April 17, 1988, Section 6 (*The Good Health Magazine*), Part 2, p. 24, col. 1; Irene Lacher, "Her Life May Read Like a Bad Soap, but Beverly Hills Broker Elaine Young Says That After Six Marriages and a Cosmetic Surgery Nightmare She's Down but Not Out," *Los Angeles Times*, April 16, 1992, p. E1, col. 2; Deborah Hastings, "Beset by Tragedy, Bad Business, Beverly Hills Real Estate Agent Goes Bust," Associated Press, March 20, 1993.

page 166: "the injection of silicone . . . a felony offense": M.J. Rapaport, M.D., C. Vinnik, M.D., and H. Zarem, M.D., "Injectable Silicone: Cause of Facial Nodules, Cellulitis, Ulceration, and Migration," *Aesthetic Plastic Surgery*, 1996, Vol. 20, pp. 267–276; Anemona Hartocollis, "What Price Beauty?" *Newsday*, June 28, 1992, p. 6.

page 167: " 'poor man's atomic bomb' ": Joan Kron, "Pretty Poison," *Allure*, January 1998, pp. 96–97; see also Norman M. Covert, *Cutting Edge: A History of Fort Detrick, Maryland* (Fort Detrick, Maryland: Public Affairs Office, U.S. Army Garrison, January 1997).

CHAPTER EIGHT: PARDON MY APPEARANCE;
I'VE JUST HAD A RUN-IN WITH A PLASTIC SURGEON

page 170: "The pleasing punishment that women bear": William Shakespeare, *The Comedy of Errors* (1592–1593), I: i.

page 170: "a husband who spent an hour holding the hand of the wrong woman": Author's interview with Nola Rocco, January 1991.

page 171: " 'assertive, perfectionist people . . . who need to feel in control of situations' ": Marcia K. Goin, Ph.D., Rodney W. Burgoyne, M.D., and John M. Goin, M.D. "Face-Lift Operation: The Patient's Secret Motivations and Reactions to Informed Consent," *Plastic and Reconstructive Surgery*, September 1976, Vol. 58, No. 3, pp. 273–279.

page 172: " 'Surprise and distress' is a common reaction": Author's interview with Donna Phillips, R.N., January 1998.

page 173: " 'We call them pocketbooks' ": Author's interview with Peggy Broderick, R.N., July 1996.

page 174: "For several months after surgery": Dixie Carter, Trying to Get to Heaven: Opinions of a Tennessee Talker (New York: Simon & Schuster, 1996), p. 89.

page 176: "The academic bible on complications": Robert M. Goldwyn, M.D., ed., The Unfavorable Result of Plastic Surgery: Avoidance and Treatment, Second Edition (Boston: Little, Brown and Company, 1984).

page 177: "Face-lift connected deaths 'are few and far between' ": Author's interview with Robert M. Goldwyn, M.D., May 1996.

page 177: "I've reported on a few cosmetic surgery deaths": Joan Kron, "Death by Face-Lift," Allure, September 1992, pp. 142–145, 178, 180–81; "Appointment With Death," Allure, February 1994, pp. 102–105, 147; "Dr. Do-it-All," Allure, September 1995, pp. 200–205, 234–236; "What Can Go Wrong," Allure, September 1996, pp. 242–249.

page 177: " 'How can cosmetic surgery leave someone dead?' ": Joan Kron, "What Can Go Wrong," Allure, September 1996, pp. 242–249.

page 177: "there is no central data base of complications and deaths": Author's interview with Mark Gorney, M.D., August 1996. (Gorney is a San Francisco plastic surgeon and vice president of the Napa-based Doctors Company, a malpractice insurance carrier. "Hospitals are required to report complications to the state," he says. But an estimated 70 percent of aesthetic surgery is performed in private offices or surgicenters—"behind closed doors." Only local coroners know the cause of death but they do not keep track of postoperative deaths by cosmetic procedure. Individual studies, complete with mortality figures, are available in the medical literature.)

page 178: " 'I know they're legally obligated' ": Elizabeth Taylor, as told to Brad Darrach, "An Extraordinary Life," Life, April 1997, pp. 78–88. (Taylor said she was warned about "stroke, paralysis, loss of memory, the possibility that they might knock me off.")

page 178: "A study of twenty face-lift patients": Marcia K. Goin, Ph.D., Rodney W. Burgoyne, M.D., and John M. Goin, M.D., "Face-Lift Operation: The Patient's Secret Motivations and Reactions to Informed Consent," Plastic & Reconstructive Surgery, September 1976, Vol. 58, No. 3, pp. 273–279.

page 179: "men have a stronger blood supply": Robert M. Goldwyn, M.D., The Unfavorable Result in Plastic Surgery: Avoidance and Treatment, Second Edition (Boston: Little, Brown and Company, 1984), p. 594.

page 179: "There is no way you can prevent": Author's interview with Eugene H. Courtiss, M.D., June 1996.

page 180: "a drama that uses a woman's face-lift": Peter Hedges, Good As New, New York: MCC Theater, February 19 to March 16, 1997.

page 182: "bleeding after eyelid surgery": Author's interview with Guy Massry, M.D., June 1996.

page 182: "the risk is four one-hundreths of one percent": M. de Mere et al., "Eye Complications with the Blepharoplasty or Other Eyelid Surgery, a National Survey," *Plastic & Reconstructive Surgery,* Vol. 53, 1974. pp. 634–637.

page 182: "There have been more than seventy-five such events": Jonathan C. Lowry, M.D., and George B. Bartley, M.D., "Complications of Blepharoplasty," *Survey of Ophthalmology,* January–February, Vol. 38, No. 4, 1994, pp. 327–345.

page 182: "The most common complications": Author's interview with James Carraway, M.D., November, 1997 and January 1998. (Carraway, a Norfolk, Virginia, plastic surgeon, says he has never seen a surgical complication of blepharoplasty that could not be corrected, However, it is generally agreed that dry eye can be helped, but not cured.)

page 182: "she feels foolish, ashamed, guilty and angry": Robert M. Goldwyn, M.D., *The Patient and the Plastic Surgeon, Second Edition* (Boston: Little, Brown and Company, 1991), p. 249.

page 186: "Pamela spent the night in the hospital": Sally Bedell Smith, *Reflected Glory: The Life of Pamela Churchill Harriman* (Simon & Schuster, 1996).

page 188: "All surgical procedures": John M. Goin, M.D., Marcia K. Goin, Ph.D., John R. Lewis, Jr., M.D., "Psychological Aspects of Aesthetic Plastic Surgery," *The Art of Aesthetic Plastic Surgery, Volume 1* (Boston: Little, Brown and Company, 1989), pp. 39–47.

page 194: "A study done at Vanderbilt Medical Center": D. Leeb, M.D., D. G. Bowers, Jr., M.D., and J. B. Lynch, M.D., "Observations on the Myth of Informed Consent," *Plastic & Reconstructive Surgery,* Vol. 58., No. 3., September 1976, pp. 280–282.

page 194: "The most dangerous patient": Joan Kron, "Appointment With Death," *Allure,* February 1994, pp. 102–105, 147.

page 194: "patients who are prone to dissatisfaction": Robert M. Goldwyn, M.D., *The Patient and the Plastic Surgeon, Second Edition* (Boston: Little, Brown and Company, 1991), pp. 64–87. (Quoted with permission.)

page 196: "The opinions of others:" Ibid, p. 156.

page 197: " 'Friends' are diabolical assassins": Robert M. Goldwyn, M.D., "Someone Out There Loves You," *Plastic & Reconstructive Surgery,* March 1991, pp. 547–548.

page 198: "Nerve weakness from a facelift": Daniel C. Baker, M.D., "Deep Dissection Rhytidectomy: A Plea for Caution," *Plastic & Reconstructive Surgery,* Vol. 93, No. 7, June 1994, pp. 1498–1499.

page 199: "90 percent of patients are happy": Joan Kron, "What Can Go Wrong," *Allure,* September 1996, pp. 242–249.

CHAPTER NINE: METAMORPHOSIS—THE BUTTERFLY EMERGES

page 205: "Obviously, it's not a good thing": Dana Kennedy, "Cher Determination," *Entertainment Weekly,* May 31, 1996, p. 22.

page 205: " 'is never fully incorporated into the body image' ": John M. Goin, M.D., and Marcia K. Goin, Ph.D., "Psychological Aspects of Aesthetic Plastic Surgery," in John R. Lewis, Jr., M.D., ed., *The Art of Aesthetic Plastic Surgery* (Boston: Little, Brown and Company, 1989), pp. 39–47.

page 207: " 'trapped in the wrong face' ": Author's interview with Milton T. Edgerton, M.D., October 1995. (Also, Joan Kron, "The Man in the Mirror: Doctors Analyze the Faces of Michael Jackson," *Allure,* January 1996, pp. 116–119, 139, 140.)

page 208: " 'as long as we could safely' ": Ibid.

page 208: "cosmetic surgery makes people happier": Author's interview with Gregory L. Borah, M.D., May 1997. (Borah is the author, with Marlene Rankin, Ph.D., Arthur Perry, M.D., and Philip Wey, M.D., of "Cosmetic Surgery Improves Quality of Life," a paper presented May 3, 1997, at the meeting of American Sociey for Aesthetic Plastic Surgery, New York Hilton.)

page 208: "patients generally like their appearance": David B. Sarwer, Ph.D., and Linton A. Whitaker, M.D., "Body Image Dissatisfaction in the Aging Face Patient," 1997, presented at the American Society for Aesthetic Plastic Surgery meeting, New York, May 1997. (In this study of fifty face-lift patients, Sarwer a psychologist at the Center for Human Appearance, University of Pennsylvania, distinguishes "type-changing" procedures such as rhinoplasties or jaw revisions, which alter appearance, from "restorative" procedures like the face-lift, which returns the individual to a previous state.)

page 208: "the majority of face-lift patients are normal": Author's interview with David B. Sarwer, Ph.D., April 1997.

page 210: "talked to me about maintenance too": Joan Kron, "To Tell The Truth," *Allure,* July 1995, pp. 120–123, 131–132.

page 211: " 'The breasts are very important organs' ": Joan Kron, "The Nip-and-Tuck Career of Ivo Pitanguy," *Allure,* September 1994, pp. 194–199, 230, 231.

page 211: "broke the code of silence": Joan Kron, "To Tell the Truth," *Allure,* July 1995, pp. 120–123, 131–132.

page 212: "meeting a high school friend": Ibid.

CHAPTER TEN: IT'S YOUR DECISION

page 214: " 'the face [is the] focus of anxiety' ": Ivo Pitanguy et al., "Incisions in Primary and Secondary Rhytidoplasties," *Revista Brasileira de Cirurgia*, August 1995, Vol. 85, No. 4, pp. 165–176.

page 215: " 'the end of the taboo' ": Rochelle Udell, "Driving Innovation by Understanding Consumer Concerns," Speech to Fashion Group International, New York, August 1996.

page 215: "7 percent of cosmetic surgery patients": Author's interview with David B. Sarwer, Ph.D., May 1997.

INDEX

Advil, 181
Agins, Teri, 135–36
AIDS, 77
All Consuming Images (Ewen), 19
Allen, Don, Studio, 81–82, 83, 84
AlloDerm, 166–67
Allure, 201
  "Shopping for a New Face" article in,
    2, 3–4, 5
Allure (Vreeland), 72–73
American Association of Facial Plastic
    and Reconstructive Surgeons
    (AAFPRS), 65
American Board of Cosmetic Surgery
    (ABCS), 64
American Board of Dermatology, 64
American Board of Medical Specialties
    (ABMS), 63–64, 65
American Board of Plastic Surgery, 71,
    76
American Medical Association (AMA),
    63, 70, 72, 76
American Society for Aesthetic Plastic
    Surgery (ASAPS), 15, 65
American Society of Anesthesiologists,
    96
American Society of Plastic and
    Reconstructive Surgeons
    (ASPRS), 65, 67, 75
Anastasi, Gaspar W., 16
anatomy, 113–14, 118–20
anesthesia, 13, 94–102
  allergy to, 97
  death from, 95, 96, 97, 99
  drugs and, 92
  general, 94–97, 98, 100–101
  goals of, 98
  levels of, 98
  local, 97, 98, 99–100, 102

  monitors and, 97, 98
  twilight sleep, 95, 98, 100–101
anesthesiologists, 14, 92, 94, 97, 99,
    103–4
Ann-Margret, 48, 165
anxiety control, in anesthesia, 98, 100
Arizona discussion group, 23–24,
    27–28, 29
arnica, 8, 92–93
Aronsohn, Richard, 41
Artecoll, 162
Ashley, Franklin, 45, 48, 165
aspirin, 8, 91–92, 180–81
associations, boards, and societies, 65,
    66
Aston, Sherrell, 111, 113

Baker, Daniel C., 60, 111, 115, 198
Baker, Thomas, 131–32, 153–54, 161
Ball, Lucille, 46
Barthelmess, Richard, 148
Barton, Fritz E., Jr., 111
Beaton, Cecil, 51
Beauty Myth, The (Wolf), 33
before and after pictures, 59, 81–85,
    86
Berle, Milton, 43–44, 49
Bernhardt, Sarah, 41–42, 109
black women, aging of, 135–36
bleeding (hematoma), 14, 91, 92, 176,
    179–82
  aspirin and, 8, 91–92, 180–81
blepharoplasties, *see* eye-lifts
blood pressure, 92, 93, 100, 176, 179,
    180, 181, 182
board certification, 63–65, 66, 71–72,
    76
boards, societies, and associations, 65,
    66

Bodies: Why We Look the Way We Do (and How We Feel About It) (Glassner), 18
Borah, Gregory, 208
Botox injections, 5–6, 16, 167–68
    number performed, 16
Bowles, Camilla Parker, 26
Brando, Marlon, 43
breast surgery, 16, 45
Brice, Fanny, 42–43, 49, 70, 129
Bridges of Madison County, The (Waller), 26
Broderick, Peggy, 173–76, 180, 188, 196, 202, 203
Brody, Jane, 7
brow-lifts, 132, 133, 191–92
    coronal, 10, 133
    endoscopic, 10, 133–34, 175
    number performed, 16
Brown, Adrienne, 88–89, 177
Brown, Helen Gurley, 1, 6, 152
Browning, Norma Lee, 58, 153
Browning, Peaches, 71
bruising, 93

canthopexy, 132
carbon-dioxide (CO_2) laser resurfacing, 10, 139–40, 155–60
Carraway, James, 131
Carter, Dixie, 174
Castenares, Salvador, 130
certified registered nurse anesthetist (CRNA), 99
Challis, Beryl, 195
Charlton, Janet, 50
cheek implants, 115
chemosurgery, *see* peels
Cher, 25, 51, 205
chin:
    implants in, 60–61
    liposuctioning of, 117
Christie, Julie, 105
Cleopatra, 124–25
Cohen, Judith, 66–67
Cohen, Selwyn, 195
collagen injections, 5–6, 16, 50, 162–63

allergy to, 162–63
Artecoll, 162
autologous, 167
Dermalogen, 166
number performed, 16
Zyplast, 163
complications, 14, 172, 176–84, 199
    bleeding, *see* bleeding
    death, 14, 95, 96, 97, 99, 177
    of eye surgery, 182
    infection, 14, 158, 160, 176, 182–84
    nerve damage, 176, 198–99
computer imaging, 85
Confidential, 149
Converse, John, 46
Cooper, Gary, 46
coronal lift, 10, 133
Coronet, 151
Corrigan, Peter, 126
cosmetic surgery:
    advertisements for, 21–22
    facilities for, 13, 101–2, 171
    history and development of, 6–7
    for men, 16
    motivations for, 208–10
    number of procedures performed, 15–16
    patient psychology and, 129
    risks of, 177; *see also* complications
    role transitions and, 20
    series of events in, 103–4
    worldwide increase in, 17
    see also surgeon; *specific procedures*
Courtiss, Eugene H., 179, 199
Cox, Meg, 36
Crawford, Cindy, 21
Crawford, Joan, 43, 46
Crone, Penny, 30–31

Dallas, Buddy, 177
Davis, Bette, 46
Davis, Kathy, 14–15, 24–25, 26–27
death, 14, 177
    from anesthesia, 95, 96, 97, 99
De Desley, Jean, 148, 150, 152

dermabrasion, 139, 144, 154–55, 202
    number of procedures performed,
    16
Dermalogen, 166
dermatologists, 64–65
Devil's Candy, The (Salamon), 51
Diana, Princess, 26
Dietrich, Marlene, 39, 43, 149, 150
Diller, Phyllis, 47–48, 49, 59, 165
Dingman, Reed, 165
Dobell, Byron, 83
doctor, *see* surgeon
Dole, Bob, 25, 32
*Dolly: My Life and Other Unfinished
    Business* (Parton), 49
Dombroff, Richard, 77
Donahue, 19
Douglas, Ann, 18
Dover, Jeff, 159
drugs, 91–92
    aspirin, 8, 91–92, 180–81

Eastwood, Clint, 26
Eckersley, Rosemary, 45
Edgerton, Milton T., 207–8
Elizabeth I, Queen, 7, 17, 144
Elle, 35–36
endoscopic brow-lift, 10, 133–34,
    175
E.N.T. specialists (otolaryngologists),
    64, 65, 72
Ewen, Stuart, 19
eyelid, broken blood vessel in, 92
eye-lifts (blepharoplasties), 6, 16, 64,
    65, 130–32
    canthopexy, 132
    complications of, 182
    laser, 24, 131–32
    number performed, 16
    recovery from, 131
    transconjunctival, 131

face, anatomy of, 113–14, 118–20
face-lifts:
    anesthesia in, *see* anesthesia
    author's first, 6, 10, 11, 12, 86, 89,
    95–96, 133, 155, 194

author's second, 2, 3, 6, 9–12,
    81–82, 85, 86, 88–89, 93–96,
    104, 105–6, 120, 128, 130, 133,
    137–38, 139, 142, 168–69, 205,
    214, 216–17
author's second, day of, 9, 12–14, 17,
    19–20, 22, 170–73
author's second, recovery from,
    170–73, 176, 184–204
before and after pictures and, 59,
    81–85, 86
complications from, *see* complications
denial of, 4
drains and, 173
friends and, 196–97, 210–13
gauze-helmet dressing for, 173
history and development of, 6–7, 18,
    106–10, 111–15
hospital stay for, 14, 171, 172
liposuction in, 117; *see also*
    liposuction
longevity of, 11, 111–12, 113
mask, 113, 114
motivations for, 208–10
nonsurgical, *see* laser resurfacing;
    peels
number performed, 16
numbness following, 174–75
options in, 111–15
pain and, 98, 100, 174
peels and, 141
reconsidering, 89
recovery from, *see* recovery
risks of, 89, 177; *see also*
    complications
satisfaction with, 207–8
scheduling of, 89–90
screws in, 192
self-acceptance after, 205–7
skin and muscle lift, 112–13
skin lift, 111–12, 114
SMAS and, 113, 114, 115, 117, 118,
    119
staples in, 188, 191
surgeon for, *see* surgeon
traveling for, 86–88
see also cosmetic surgery

*Face-lifts: Everything You Always Wanted
    to Know* (Browning), 58
Faces (Lord), 150
Face Value: The Politics of Beauty (Lakoff
    and Scherr), 85
Fame in the Twentieth Century (James),
    41
Feldman, Joel, 117–18
fingernails, 14
Fitzpatrick, Richard, 157
Flaubert, Gustave, 81
Flowers, Robert, 130, 132
Foltyn, Jacque Lynn, 33, 125
Fonda, Jane, 51
food, 13
Ford, Eileen, 166
Fournier, Pierre, 126
Fowles, Jib, 44, 50, 51
Fox, James, 127
frown muscles, 134
Frühwald, Victor, 108

Gable, Clark, 46
Gabor, Eva, 50
Gabor, Jolie, 46, 165–66
Gabor, Zsa Zsa, 50
Galenti, Cora, 149–50, 152, 153, 154
Gamson, Joshua, 52
Garbo, Greta, 41
Getting Over Getting Older (Pogrebin),
    31
Gillies, Harold Delf, 105
Glamour, 76
Glassner, Barry, 17–18
Gleason, Jackie, 49
Goin, John and Marcia, 27, 178–79,
    184, 188, 205–6
Goldwyn, Robert M., 38, 56, 176,
    177, 182, 194, 196–97
Good Housekeeping, 72
Gordon, Howard, 153–54
Gordon, Martin, 99–100
Gore-Tex implants, 57, 161
Gorney, Mark, 194
Grace, Princess, 150
Gradé, Arthur, 146–48, 150–51, 152,
    154
Grey, Jennifer, 121

Griffith, Melanie, 51
Guggenheim, Peggy, 108
Guglielmi, Albert, 43
Gunter, Jack, 120–21
Gurdin, Michael, 44, 45, 46

hairdressers, 58
Halton, Eugene, 158
Hamra, Sam T., 113, 115
Harper's Bazaar, 47, 72
Harriman, Pamela, 51, 186–87
Havoc, June, 43
hematoma, *see* bleeding
Hobson, Irehne, 147, 148
Hoefflin, Steven M., 41, 103
Hollander, Eugen, 106–7
Hughes, Howard, 150
Hutton, Barbara, 46
hypertrophic scars, 136, 155, 160

Ideal Husband, The (Wilde), 126
Illouz, Yves-Gérard, 53, 116–17
Imber, Gerald, 115
Importance of Being Beautiful, The
    (Foltyn), 33, 125
Independent Woman, 70
infection, 14, 176, 182–84
    laser and, 158, 160
Iverson, Ronald E., 67

Jackson, Michael, 41, 50, 128, 208
James, Clive, 41
job market, 20–21
Joseph, Jacques, 108, 128–29
jowls, liposuctioning of, 117

Kamer, Frank, 49, 115
Kane, Michael, 59
keloids, 1, 136
Kelsen, Venner, 151–52, 154
Klein, Arnold, 161
Knipper, Patrick, 119–20

Ladies Home Journal, 34, 47, 145, 164
La Gassé, Antoinette, 148–49, 153
Lakoff, Robin Tolmach, 85
Lamarr, Hedy, 43
Lambert, Eleanor, 75

Lamont, Edward, 43
Lancaster, Burt, 43
Lange, Jessica, 49
Lansbury, Angela, 25
laser blepharoplasty (eye-lift), 24,
    131–32
laser resurfacing, 131, 156, 160–61
    carbon-dioxide (CO$_2$), 10, 139–40,
        155–60
    cautions with, 158–59, 160
    Erbium, 140, 160
    infection and, 158, 160
    number of procedures performed,
        16
    scarring from, 158, 160, 202
    swelling from, 159–60
Leach, Robin, 40
Leaf, Norman, 135, 136
Lemmon, Mark, 113
Leno, Jay, 25, 32
Lexer, Erich, 107
Lewis, Wendy, 79
lidocaine, 99, 100
life expectancy, 20
lip, Gore-Tex enhancement of, 57,
    161
lip, upper, peel on, 139, 142–43,
    154–55, 160, 168–69
liposuction, 16, 19, 53, 65, 99
    of chin and jowls, 117
    development of, 116–17
    number of procedures performed,
        16
Lister, Joseph, 144–45
Litton, Clyde, 154
Longevity, 84
Look, 43–44
Lord, Shirley, 150
Lorenc, Paul, 201

McCall's, 47
McCarthy, Joseph G., 117
McCracken, Grant, 11, 21, 26, 122
McDowell, Frank, 65
McKinney, Peter, 112
McLellan, Diana, 25, 37
Mademoiselle, 76
Makeover Miracles (Merron), 43

Manhattan Eye, Ear & Throat Hospital
    (MEETH), 2, 3, 82, 96, 173
Manual of Chemical Peels (Rubin), 155
Maschek, Miriam and Francis,
    152–53, 154
mask-lift, 113, 114
Massry, Guy, 182
Matarasso, Alan, 137
Meisel, Steven, 25
Menkes, Suzy, 50–51
Merron, Michael, 43
Mies van der Rohe, Ludwig, 81
Miller, Charles Conrad, 107–8
Miller, Lois Mattox, 70–71
Mitchum, Robert, 43
Mitz, Vladimir, 111, 112, 113, 118
moles, 135
Monroe, Marilyn, 44, 45
Moore, Pat, 12
Morello, Daniel, 93
More Than Just a Pretty Face (Rees), 28
Morini, Simona, 73
movie stars, 39–46, 49–52, 59
Murray, Mae, 44, 147

nasal-labial fold, 161
neck, 116, 119
nerve damage, 176, 198–99
Newsweek, 76
New York, 27
New York Post, 121
New York Times, 12, 42
New York Times Magazine, 75–76
Noël, Suzanne, 109–10
nose:
    of Cleopatra, 124–25
    dropping of, 120
nose surgery (rhinoplasty), 10–11, 16,
    64, 120–29
    adjustment period following, 127
    dissatisfaction with, 194–95
    history of, 122–24
    number of procedures performed, 16
    repair and reconstruction, 122–24
Nyberg, Tom, 97–98, 101

Oberon, Merle, 43, 45
Onassis, Jacqueline Kennedy, 25, 82

ophthalmologists, 64
otolaryngologists (E.N.T. specialists),
    64, 65, 72
Owsley, John Q., 113, 114

pacemakers, 102
pain control, 98, 100, 174
    in peels, 152
Paley, Babe, 71, 112
Pangman, John, 44–45
paraffin, 163–64
Parker, Dorothy, 25, 42, 129
Parker, Jean, 149–50
Parton, Dolly, 49
Patient and Plastic Surgery, The
    (Goldwyn), 38
Patterson, Ethel Lloyd, 34–35
Pearson, Wayne, 84
peels (chemosurgery), 16, 21, 65, 131,
    139–55
    face-lifts and, 141
    history and development of, 7,
        143–54
    lip, 139, 142–43, 154–55, 160,
        168–69
    number performed, 16
    pain control in, 152
    phenol, 139, 144–45, 146, 147,
        149, 150, 152–54, 155
    scarring from, 202
    skin shrinkage and, 161
    TCA, 10, 140–41, 155, 160, 202
    see also dermabrasion; laser
        resurfacing
People, 49
Perelman, S. J., 108
Peyronie, Martine, 113
phenol peels, 139, 144–45, 146, 147,
    149, 150, 152–54, 155
Phillips, Donna, 172, 190
Pitanguy, Ivo, 73–76, 211, 214
Pius XII, Pope, 150–51
plastic surgeon, see surgeon
plastic surgery, see cosmetic surgery
Plenitude (McCracken), 26
Pogrebin, Letty Cottin, 31–32
Presley, Elvis, 127

Presley, Lisa Marie, 50
Price, David, 81, 82
Primetime Live, 159

Quinn, Jane Bryant, 33

Raphael, Sally Jesse, 7
Recamier, Julie de, 85–86
recovery, 2, 8, 32, 87–88, 170–76,
    184–204
    of author, from second lift, 170–73,
        176, 184–204
    emotions in, 188
    from eye-lift, 131
    personality and, 184
    time for, 87, 88, 175
    see also complications
Rees, Thomas, 28, 36, 46, 71, 74, 75,
    76, 77, 112, 137
Reshaping the Female Body (Davis),
    14–15
Revolution From Within (Steinem), 33
rhinoplasty, see nose surgery
Ribes, Jacqueline de, 51
Ristow, Brunno, 112
Rivera, Geraldo, 157–58
Rivers, Joan, 11, 49
Roberts, Thomas, III, 156, 159, 160
Rocco, Nola, 170
Roe, John, 128
Rogers, Blair, 106
Roseanne, 49
Royal, Christine, 27
Rubin, Mark, 155

Salamon, Julie, 51
Sanders, Clinton, 12
Sarwer, David B., 208–9
scars, 1, 135–38, 202
    hypertrophic, 136, 155, 160
    keloid, 1, 136
    from laser resurfacing, 158, 160,
        202
    in people of color, 135, 136
    position of, 136–37
Schenk, Joe, 43
Scherr, Raquel L., 85

Schireson, Henry Junius, 70, 71
Schouten, John W., 20
Scottsdale, Ariz., 23–24, 27–28, 29
Seifert, Lawrence N., 81, 101
Seldes, Gilbert, 9
Self, 215
Shakespeare, William, 170
Shaw, Sarah (Antoinette La Gassé),
    148–49, 153
Sheehy, Gail, 1
Sheen, Jack, 127
Shue, Elisabeth, 49
Silent Passage, The: Menopause
    (Sheehy), 1
silicone, liquid, 44–45, 161–62,
    164–66
Silver, L. David, 96
Simpson, Wallis, Duchess of Windsor,
    51
Sitwell, Osbert, 35
skin peels, *see* peels
Skoog, Törd, 112–13, 114, 115
sleep:
    in anesthesia, 98
    after lift, 176
SMAS (superficial musculo-
    aponeurotic system), 113, 114,
    115, 117, 118, 119
Smith, Liz, 26
Smith, Sally Bedell, 51, 186–87
smoking, 91
societies, boards, and associations, 65,
    66
Sorel, Cecile, 109–10
Stallone, Jacqueline, 154
Star, 50
Steinem, Gloria, 1, 6, 33, 47
Stone, Phillip A., 146
Stuzin, James M., 93
surgeon(s):
    artistic credentials of, 66
    asking questions of, 90
    author's choosing of, 53–56, 61–63,
        67–69, 77–80
    board-certified, 63–65, 66, 71–72,
        76
    choosing of, 53–80

matchmakers and, 66–67
named in magazines, 59–60
operating privileges and, 65–66
unscrupulous, 7, 69–71, 76–77
Swanson, Gloria, 41, 150

Tagliacozzi, Gaspare, 32, 34,
    123–24
Taylor, Elizabeth, 46, 173, 178, 199
TCA (tri-chloroacetic acid) peels, 10,
    140–41, 155, 160, 202
TC-bleph (transconjunctival
    blepharoplasty), 131
television, 19, 45
Terino, Edward, 50
*Terrible Honesty: Mongrel Manhattan in
    the 1920s* (Douglas), 18
Tessier, Paul, 113, 114
Thomas, Jacques, 152
tragus, 136–37
Trotta, Geri, 43–44, 47, 72
Turner, Lana, 43, 151
20/20, 19
twilight sleep, 95, 98, 100–101

Udell, Rochelle, 215
*Unfavorable Result of Plastic Surgery,
    The* (Goldwyn, ed.), 176
USA Today, 27

Valentino, Rudolf, 43
Vandermeer, Nienke, 27
vitamins, 92
Vogue, 72–73, 113, 150, 164, 165
Vreeland, Diana, 72–73

Waller, Robert James, 26
Wall Street Journal, 16, 19, 20–21,
    135
Walters, Barbara, 152
Washingtonian, 25, 37
Wayne, John, 43, 48
Weathers, Seaborn, 123
Webber, Meridyth, 186
Weir, Robert Fulton, 128
Wells, Linda, 3
West, Mae, 148, 149

Wheeland, Ronald G., 158
Wilde, Oscar, 126
Willi, Charles H., 109
Williams, John, 50
Wolf, Naomi, 33
Working Woman, 33

Young, Elaine, 166
Yousif, John N., 113, 114
Youth Corridor, The (Imber), 115

Zarem, Harvey A., 84
Zyplast, 163